D1173584

The Institutional Review Board
Member Handbook

Also of interest

Institutional Review Board: Management and Function,
Amdur and Bankert, Ed., © 2002 Jones and Bartlett
Publishers. ISBN 0-7637-1686-3

Study Guide for the Institutional Review Board:
Management and Function, Kornetsky, © 2003 Jones and
Bartlett Publishers. ISBN 0-7637-2259-6

The Institutional Review Board Member Handbook

Robert J. Amdur, M.D.
University of Florida College of Medicine

JONES AND BARTLETT PUBLISHERS
Sudbury, Massachusetts
BOSTON   TORONTO   LONDON   SINGAPORE

World Headquarters
Jones and Bartlett Publishers
40 Tall Pine Drive
Sudbury, MA 01776
978-443-5000
info@jbpub.com
www.jbpub.com

Jones and Bartlett Publishers Canada
2406 Nikanna Road
Mississauga, ON L5C 2W6
CANADA

Jones and Bartlett Publishers International
Barb House, Barb Mews
London W6 7PA
UK

Library of Congress Cataloging-in-Publication Data

Amdur, Robert J.
    Institutional review board member handbook / Robert J. Amdur.
        p. cm.
    Includes index.
    ISBN 0-7637-2257-X
Institutional review boards (Medicine)—Handbooks, manuals, etc.
I. Title.

R852.5 .A463 2003
610'.7'2—dc21

                                                    2002034162

Production Credits
Acquisitions Editor: Penny M. Glynn
Production Manager: Amy Rose
Editorial Assistant: Karen Zuck
Associate Production Editor: Karen C. Ferreira
Senior Marketing Manager: Alisha Weisman
Marketing Associate: Joy Stark-Vancs
Manufacturing and Inventory Coordinator: Amy Bacus
Cover Design: Philip Regan
Composition: Chiron, Inc.
Printing and Binding: United Graphics Incorporated
Cover Printing: United Graphics Incorporated

Printed in the United States of America
06 05 04   10 9 8 7 6 5

CONTENTS

CONTRIBUTORS

Robert J. Amdur, M.D.
Professor
Radiation Oncology
University of Florida College of Medicine
Gainesville, FL

Elizabeth A. Bankert, M.A.
Director
Committee for the Protection of Human Subjects
Dartmouth College
Hanover, NH

Joseph S. Brown, Ph.D.
Associate Professor
Psychology
University of Nebraska at Omaha
Omaha, NE

Marianne M. Elliott, M.S., C.I.P.
Director
Office for Protection of Research Subjects
University of Illinois at Chicago
Chicago, IL

Richard B. Ferrell, M.D.
Associate Professor
Psychiatry
Dartmouth Hitchcock Medical Center
Lebanon, NH

Dean R. Gallant, A.B.
Director, Science Center and Executive Officer
Committee on the Use of Human Subjects in Research
Harvard University
Cambridge, MA

Bruce G. Gordon, M.D.
IRB Co-Chair and Associate Professor
Pediatrics
University of Nebraska Medical Center
Omaha, NE

Karen M. Hansen, B.A.
Director
Institutional Review Office
Fred Hutchinson Cancer Research Center
Seattle, WA

Rachel Homer, B.S.
IRB Coordinator
Clinical Investigation
Children's Hospital
Boston, MA

Jay G. Hull, Ph.D.
Professor
Psychological and Brain Sciences
Dartmouth College
Hanover, NH

Thomas G. Keens, M.D.
Chair
Committee on Clinical Investigations (IRB)
Children's Hospital
Los Angeles, CA

Linda J. Kobokovich, M.Sc.N., R.N.
Director of Nursing Practice
Dartmouth Hitchcock Medical Center
Lebanon, NH

Susan Z. Kornetsky, M.P.H., C.I.P.
Director
Clinical Research Compliance
Children's Hospital
Boston, MA

Gail Kotulak, B.S.
IRB Administrator
University of Nebraska Medical Center
Omaha, NE

Christopher J. Kratochvil, M.D.
Vice-Chair, IRB and Assistant Professor
Psychiatry
University of Nebraska Medical Center
Omaha, NE

Rachel Krebs, B.S.
Senior Coordinator
Clinical Investigations
Children's Hospital
Boston, MA

Linda Medwar, B.S.
Senior IRB Coordinator
Children's Hospital
Boston, MA

Matthew Miller, M.D., M.P.H., Sc.D.
Associate Director
Health Policy and Management
Harvard Injury Control Research Center, Harvard
School of Public Health
Brookline, MA

Daniel K. Nelson, M.S., C.I.P.
Associate Professor and Director
Human Research Studies, School of Medicine
University of North Carolina at Chapel Hill
Chapel Hill, NC

Robert M. Nelson, M.D., Ph.D.
Associate Professor
Anesthesia and Pediatrics
Children's Hospital of Philadelphia
University of Pennsylvania School of Medicine
Philadelphia, PA

Ernest D. Prentice, Ph.D.
Associate Dean of Research, Professor, Co-Chair, IRB
and Associate Vice-Chancellor for Academic Affairs
and Regulatory Compliance
Anatomy
University of Nebraska Medical Center
Omaha, NE

Thomas Puglisi, Ph.D.
PricewaterhouseCoopers
Bethesda, MD

Michele Russell-Einhorn, J.D.
PricewaterhouseCoopers
Bethesda, MD

Laurie B. Slone
Graduate Student
Psychologic and Brain Sciences
Dartmouth College
Hanover, NH

DEDICATION

To IRB members everywhere who understand that
protecting the rights and welfare of research subjects
requires a commitment to higher ideals, the motivation
to evaluate complex issues, and the courage to make
unpopular decisions.

Let us all remember that a slower progress in the con-
quest of disease would not threaten society, grievous as
it is to those who deplore that particular disease be not
yet conquered but that, society would indeed be threatened by the erosion of those moral values whose loss,
possibly caused by too ruthless a pursuit of scientific
progress, would make its most dazzling triumphs not
worth having.*

*Jonas H. 1970. "Philosophical Reflections on Experimenting with
Human Subjects." In *Experimentation with Human Subjects*, edited by
Paul A. Freund. New York: George Braziller, pp. 16–17.

INTRODUCTION

ROBERT J. AMDUR

Congratulations on your appointment to the Institutional Review Board (IRB). Service on the IRB is said to be one of the best forms of continuing education available to a person who is interested in medicine or the social sciences. You will be exposed to new ideas in a wide range of scientific fields, and the decisions you make and the opinions you bring to the IRB will have implications both for the people who conduct research activities as well as those who participate in them.

As an IRB member, your mission is to help researchers conduct important studies in a way that protects the rights and welfare of the research participants. People who do not understand how the IRB should function may think that making IRB determinations is a simple job that requires little more than common sense and good intentions. This is often not the case. As you learn more about research ethics and research regulation, you will understand that many research projects present ethical issues that are not straightforward to recognize or resolve. Common sense and good intentions are required for you to function effectively on the IRB, but these qualities are not enough. You also have to have a structured approach to evaluating the ethics of a research protocol and a clear understanding of the fundamental principles that you should use to determine how to vote on specific studies. This handbook will give you this information. Again, congratulations on your appointment to the IRB.

PART 1

BACKGROUND INFORMATION

C H A P T E R 1-1

THE PURPOSE OF THIS HANDBOOK

ROBERT J. AMDUR

IS THIS HANDBOOK FOR YOU?

This handbook is written specifically for the voting members of an Institutional Review Board (IRB).

WHAT WILL THIS BOOK DO FOR YOU?

This handbook explains the background of the IRB system, what IRB discussions are suppose to focus on, what IRB members should do before each IRB meeting, and how members should conduct themselves during the meeting. It also summarizes basic guidelines for evaluating specific kinds of studies.

WILL THIS HANDBOOK TELL YOU EVERYTHING YOU NEED TO KNOW?

No. This handbook provides the basic information that you need to do a good job as an IRB member. Research ethics and research regulation are complex fields with constantly changing standards and levels of complexity. You will frequently encounter situations that are not explained in this book. Continuing education is required for you to keep up with important and evolving IRB issues.

WHAT EDUCATIONAL MATERIALS SHOULD YOU REVIEW BESIDES THIS HANDBOOK?

This handbook gives you the basic information you need to be an excellent IRB member. There are numerous other educational publications that explain IRB issues in more detail. A detailed list of educational resources is presented in Part 4 of this handbook. However, there are two resources that you should focus on. (Before ordering either of these yourself, you may want to ask your IRB administrative director to order them, or there may be copies available for you to borrow.)

The first resource is a videotape called *Protecting Human Subjects* that the Office of Human Research Protection will send you at no charge. This video is an excellent review of the history of the IRB system and the fundamental ethical principles that you need to use when evaluating specific research projects. It is really worth looking at. Here is the information needed to order this excellent educational resource:

Videotape Series: *Protecting Human Subjects*

Ordering Information: There is no charge for this videotape. Send requestor name, title, institution name, address, and telephone number via letter to Gail Carter, Program Assistant, Office for Human Research Protections, Tower Building, 1101 Wootton Parkway, Suite 200, Rockville, MD 20852, or FAX your request to (301) 402-0527 (ATTN: Gail Carter), or e-mail your request to gcarter@osophs.dhhs.gov.

The second resource is a comprehensive textbook on IRB issues called *Institutional Review Board: Management and Function*, written by many experts in the field of research regulation. Although the book covers many areas that will not be of interest to IRB members and may not be something that every IRB member will find useful, it is the place to go if you want to learn more about IRB issues, including a comprehensive list of other books, journals, and websites that cover topics that are applicable to the IRB. Here is the information you will need to order the textbook:

Institutional Review Board: Management and Function

Edited by Robert J. Amdur and Elizabeth A. Bankert
  Published by Jones and Bartlett, Sudbury, MA,
  January 2002 ISBN 0763716863
  Online ordering information:
  http://catalog.jbpub.com/detail.cfm?i=1686-3
  Cost: approximately $125

YOUR MISSION ON THE IRB

ROBERT J. AMDUR

WHAT IS YOUR ROLE AS AN IRB MEMBER?

The mission of the Institutional Review Board (IRB) is to protect the rights and welfare of research subjects. Every decision made on the IRB should be driven by this specific goal. Although you will encounter many situations where it will be easy to get distracted by issues that are not directly related to the protection of research subjects, resist this temptation. IRB review is a specialized process that is designed to evaluate the ethics of research involving human subjects. Because this is such a complicated job, anything that distracts you from your fundamental goal will likely compromise the quality of your work on the IRB. To help you focus your efforts when evaluating a research protocol, it may be useful to ask yourself this question:

IS A CHANGE IN THE RESEARCH PROTOCOL LIKELY TO IMPROVE THE WELFARE OF RESEARCH SUBJECTS TO A MEANINGFUL DEGREE?

If your answer to this question is "no," then you should approve the research proposal without changing it. If your answer to this question is "yes," then you should not approve the research plan as proposed.

WHAT IS AN IRB?

The IRB is a committee whose primary responsibility is to protect the rights and welfare of research subjects and to function as a kind of ethics committee focusing on what is right or wrong and on what is desirable or undesirable. The IRB is thus required to make judgments about what individuals and groups ought to do and how they ought to do it.

The Institutional Review Board is an American organization. In other countries terms such as "Research Ethics Committee" or "Ethical Review Board" are used to describe a committee that evaluates the ethical aspects of research involving human subjects.

There is currently no law or national directive in the United States that requires research to be reviewed in a uniform way regardless of researcher affiliation or funding source. For this reason there are many situations in which research with human subjects is conducted without approval from any type of ethics committee. Similarly, when an organization does set up a system to review the ethics of research proposals, there are many situations in which the review process and approval standards may be customized without regard for external requirements.

In the United States the only place that an IRB is formally defined is in the code of federal regulations. We will talk briefly about federal regulations later, but at this point it is sufficient to think of the federal regulations as the rules that tell the different agencies in our federal government how they must operate. Both the U.S. Department of Health and Human Services and the Food and Drug Administration have established regulations that require IRB approval to conduct research that is funded by or otherwise subject to the authority of these federal agencies. In this setting the federal regulations present a detailed set of standards that define an IRB and establish the policy and procedures by which an IRB must operate.

For the purposes of this handbook, the reference standard for IRB practice is U.S. federal research regulations. This handbook will not discuss alternatives to the federal IRB system.

CHAPTER 1-3

A BRIEF HISTORY OF THE IRB SYSTEM

ROBERT J. AMDUR

As recently as 1950, the federal government had a relatively minor role in regulating research conduct. There were no federal regulations that required IRB approval to conduct research involving human subjects in most settings. Policy and procedures for IRB review of research had not been formally defined. Ethical standards for conducting research with human subjects were not uniformly applied or accepted.

Today the situation is very different. The federal government is extensively involved in regulating almost all aspects of the research process. Most federal agencies have adopted regulations that require IRB approval to conduct research that is under their authority. The policy and procedures described in the federal regulations apply to both biomedical and social science research and have established the modern IRB system for monitoring research conduct. At the time of the writing of this handbook in late 2002, there wss a bill before the U.S. Congress that would further expand the authority of the federal government by elevating federal research regulations to the level of a federal law.

How did we go from so little to so much regulation in a relatively short period of time? The answer to this question is the history of the modern IRB system. It is a fascinating story that involves the national media, community activism, high-powered science, and big-government politics. Clearly, a separate book could be written about this subject, but only a cursory review is within the scope of this handbook. For more information on the history of research regulation, the reader is referred to the videotape described in Chapter 1-1 and to the bible of research ethics, *The Ethics and Regulation of Clinical Research* by Robert Levine described in Chapter 4-5.

However, because IRB members will function more effectively if they understand the major events that have shaped current IRB guidelines, the remainder of this chapter will briefly describe the main milestones in the history of research regulation in the United States.

1948: THE NUREMBERG CODE

The Nuremberg Trials were conducted at the end of World War II to bring justice to Nazi leaders who had committed crimes against humanity in their treatment of civilian prisoners under their control. A major portion of the trials was devoted to the case of Nazi physicians who had forced prisoners to undergo horrifying procedures for research purposes. To make the case of crimes against humanity, the prosecutors had to argue that the Nazi defendants conducted research in ways that violated the fundamental ethical standards of civilized society. However, at the time that these trials were conducted there was no established law, regulation, code, or formal document that defined the ethical standards for conducting research with human subjects in a way that was directly applicable to the Nuremberg case. As part of the proceedings at Nuremberg, the prosecution issued what is now referred to as the Nuremberg Code—a document that articulated the basic requirements for conducting research in a way that respects the fundamental rights of research subjects. The full text of the Nuremberg Code is reproduced in *Institutional Review Board: Management and Function*, the textbook mentioned in Chapter 1-1. The code can also be read online at http://www.ushmm.org/research/doctors/Nuremberg_Code.htm.

The Nuremberg Code articulated ethical standards that have been incorporated into most subsequent ethical codes (such as the Declaration of Helsinki, described below) and to a large degree in federal research regulations. The basic elements of the Nuremberg Code are the requirement for voluntary and informed consent, a favorable risk/benefit analysis, and the right to withdraw without penalty. IRB members are encouraged to read the Nuremberg Code and to refer to this document when evaluating specific IRB questions.

1955: THE WICHITA JURY STUDY

In the early 1950s social science researchers at the University of Chicago directed a study to better understand the decision-making process of jurors in criminal trials. A motivation for this study was the concern that showmanship on the part of trial attorneys might have a major influence on the jury verdict. One can only imagine the cynical comments that this kind of discussion would elicit today!

The study involved audiotaping jury deliberations in criminal trials in Wichita, Kansas. To avoid influencing their behavior, the jurors where not informed that they were subjects of a research project or that their discussions would be recorded. The study was completed as planned, and the results were presented in respected academic forums. Public reaction to the Wichita Jury Study was not favorable. The study was initially criticized in local newspapers, and it soon became the focus of national discussion. The issue was not the details of this particular study but the basic problem of deceiving people for research purposes in a setting where privacy and confidentiality were critically important. Congressional hearings were held on the subject.

Eventually Congress passed a federal law that prohibited the recording of jury deliberations in any setting. There are two main reasons that the events that followed the Wichita study are milestones in the history of research regulation in the United States:

1. The legislation that was passed in response to the Wichita study marks the first time that the actions of well-meaning researchers resulted in the establishment of federal guidelines to protect the public from exploitation.

2. The Wichita study was the first event that focused national attention on the concept that there are settings where important research questions cannot be answered without compromising the integrity of important social institutions. The scientific importance of the Wichita study was never an issue. The rationale for congressional action in this case was that the integrity of the jury process requires an environment where jurors have confidence that their deliberations are not being observed by outside parties. If our society allowed a jury deliberation to be recorded for research purposes, it might compromise all future jury deliberations.

1962: THE THALIDOMIDE EXPERIENCE

Thalidomide is a drug that was used in the 1950s to treat a variety of unpleasant symptoms associated with pregnancy. At the time that thalidomide was being used in the United States, it was not standard practice to inform patients of the investigational nature of medications that were still in the testing phase of the regulatory process. After large numbers of pregnant women were treated with thalidomide, it became clear that this drug caused severe growth deformities in their infants. Public outrage over the situation led to an amendment to the Food, Drug, and Cosmetic Act that basically required investigators to obtain informed consent from potential subjects before administering investigational medications. This legislation thus became a milestone in the history of research regulation in the United States—the first major step in the process of using a federal agency to establish and enforce specific ethical standards for the conduct of research.

1964: NIH ETHICS COMMITTEE

In the mid-1950s the Clinical Research Center (CRC) at the National Institutes of Health was created to oversee the conduct of clinical research. CRC policy required that all research conducted at this facility be approved by a committee focusing on ethical issues. The same process was going on less formally at both public and private institutions all over the country, where local investigators saw the need for a formal review of the ethical implications of research activity. A milestone in the use of ethical review committees came in 1964 when NIH director James Shannon established a policy that required an ethics committee to review all research funded by the Public Health Service. As part of this effort, Dr. Shannon articulated the need for a formal process to ensure that all research involving human subjects was to be conducted according to a uniform set of ethical standards.

1964: THE WORLD MEDICAL ASSOCIATION DECLARATION OF HELSINKI

In 1964 the World Medical Association met in Helsinki, Finland, to draft the Declaration of Helsinki, a document that would build on the Nuremberg Code of 1948 to describe the standards of ethical research involving human subjects. The association has met many times since 1964 to reaffirm or make minor revisions to the declaration. Last revised in 2000, the Declaration of Helsinki basically consists of the standards described in the Nuremberg Code plus statements that make two key points:

- That the interests of the subject should always be given a higher priority than those of society.

- That every subject in clinical research should get the best known treatment.

IRB members are encouraged to read the Declaration of Helsinki and to apply the stated principles when making IRB determinations. The latest version of this document is included in *Institutional Review Board: Management and Function*, the textbook mentioned in Chapter 1-1. It may also be read online at http://www.wma.net/e/policy/17-c_e.html.

1966: THE ETHICS OF CLINICAL RESEARCH AND THE *NEW ENGLAND JOURNAL OF MEDICINE*

In 1966 the *New England Journal of Medicine* published an article entitled "Ethics of Clinical Research" by Henry Beecher, a senior member of the Department of Anesthesiology at Harvard Medical School. In this article Dr. Beecher described twenty-two studies that had been conducted by respected investigators and recently published in prestigious medical journals. For each of these studies, Beecher explained why the study was unethical based on fundamental principles such as lack of informed consent and increased risk to subjects. His conclusion about the status of medical research in the United States left no room for misunderstanding:

> What seem to be breeches of ethical conduct in experimentation are by no means rare but are almost, one fears, universal.... A particularly pernicious myth is the one that depends on the view that ends justify means. A study is ethical or not at its inception...whoever gave the investigator the godlike right of choosing martyrs?

Beecher's article is a milestone in the history of research ethics because it was an unprecedented attempt by a respected member of the research community to focus attention on the need to improve the ethical standards for conducting clinical research in this country. An article this length is rarely seen in the medical literature today. While it is not essential that IRB members read this article to function effectively on the IRB, doing so will help give them the confidence and insight needed to question accepted research procedures. It is also interesting reading in its own right. The reference for the Beecher article is *New England Journal of Medicine* 274 (1966): 1354–1360.

1973: CONGRESSIONAL HEARINGS ON THE QUALITY OF HEALTH CARE AND HUMAN EXPERIMENTATION

In 1973 Senator Edward Kennedy directed a series of congressional hearings in response to public concern about ethical problems in the way medical research was being conducted in this country. The main catalyst for conducting these hearings was public reaction to a federally sponsored study on the natural history of syphilis that has become known as the Tuskegee Syphilis Experiment. However, it is probably more accurate to view this period of congressional activity as the result of a long string of high-profile events involving both biomedical and social science research. The remainder of this subsection briefly describes some of the events that were pivotal in focusing public attention on issues related to research ethics. The purpose here is to give IRB members a feel for the issues congressional representatives were thinking about when they debated the need for extending federal oversight of research involving human subjects. It is important to note that this is only a partial list and that many important efforts and details are not described.

Willowbrook Hepatitis Studies

In the 1950s a series of studies were done to understand issues related to the transmission of the hepatitis virus in retarded children who where residents in the Willowbrook state school, an extended care facility in New York state. Because a high percentage of residents contracted hepatitis during their time at Willowbrook, there was no question about the importance of understanding more about the mode of transmission of the hepatitis virus in this population. The aspect of this research that generated debate in both the national media and professional journals was a study design that involved intentionally infecting healthy children with hepatitis by feeding them a solution made from the feces of children with active hepatitis.

Jewish Chronic Disease Hospital Studies

In the 1960s a series of experiments were performed on chronically ill, mostly demented patients in the Jewish Chronic Disease Hospital in New York City. All of the subjects had illnesses that compromised their immune system. The purpose of the research was to determine how a weakened immune system influenced the spread of cancer. To evaluate this issue, live cancer cells were injected into the bloodstream of the subjects.

Milgram Studies of Obedience to Authority

In the early 1960s psychologist Stanley Milgram conducted a series of studies that continue to generate controversy today. The studies were designed in the aftermath of World War II when the world was trying understand the acts of genocide that occurred during the Holocaust. The basic purpose of the Milgram studies was to understand why people follow the directions of authority figures even when they are told to do things that are cruel or unethical.

Basically the experiment involved subjects who were deceived into thinking that they were helping with a study to evaluate the role of negative reinforcement on learning. The subject was instructed to deliver an electric shock when a person who was playing the role of the "learner" answered a question incorrectly. As the study progressed, the person who was actually the study subject was ordered to give progressively stronger punishment shocks. More than half of the subjects eventually delivered what they thought were high-intensity, potentially lethal shocks in spite of expressions of serious distress on the part of the person who was playing the role of the "learner." After completion of the study, the subjects were "debriefed" about the true purpose of the study, the nature of the deception, and potential implications of their behavior. Many of the subjects experienced extreme psychological distress after understanding the level of cruelty of their actions.

San Antonio Contraception Study

In the early 1970s a study was conducted in a contraception clinic in San Antonio, Texas, that evaluated the efficacy of different kinds of female contraceptive pills. The clinic served predominantly indigent patients who had no other place to go for contraceptive advice or medication. The study involved randomizing subjects between active contraceptive and placebo pills. The women were not informed that they were the subjects of this type of research or that they might be receiving inactive medication. As expected, there was a high number of unplanned pregnancies in the placebo group.

Tearoom Trade Study

In the early 1970s social scientist Laud Humphries conducted a study of homosexual behavior in public restrooms. Dr. Humphries was able to function as a "watch queen" outside public restrooms where people gathered to engage in anonymous homosexual activity. Humphries recorded the license numbers and other identifying information from the people who came for these kinds of interactions and used this information to obtain names and addresses. He went to the homes of his study subjects and presented himself as an interviewer to collect information about the subject's background and family life. Many of the subjects were living with their family in a situation where it would be devastating to reveal information about homosexual activity. At no time did the subjects understand that they were participating in research. In published reports of this study, the level of detail was such that the identity of some of the subjects became known.

Tuskegee Syphilis Study

Between 1932 and 1972, the U.S. Public Health Service funded a study to evaluate the natural history of untreated syphilis in human beings. When this study was initiated, its basic concept was considered scientifically important and ethically justifiable because there was no effective treatment for this devastating disease. In retrospect, the main problem with this research was that the subject population was one of the most vulnerable in our society—approximately 300 indigent, uneducated, African-American sharecroppers in Macon County in Alabama who were known to have syphilis. This study is now infamous in the world of research ethics and research regulation. It is usually referred to as the Tuskegee Study, the Tuskegee Syphilis Study, or simply Tuskegee in reference to the city in Alabama where the study was headquartered.

The subjects of the Tuskegee Study did not have a meaningful understanding of their condition or the nature of the research that was being conducted. Although deception may not have been intentional on the part of the investigators, the reality is that the subjects thought they were receiving beneficial medical care and did not understand that they were participating in research that was designed specifically to observe the course of their illness. Participants were subjected to various tests and procedures—such as spinal taps—that were done solely for research purposes. The subjects were followed without treatment for many years after penicillin became widely available and was known to be beneficial in the treatment of syphilis. The study was stopped in 1972 after high-profile stories in the national media generated public outrage over the blatant exploitation of this vulnerable segment of our society.

The fact that the Tuskegee Study was directed by the federal government over such a long period of time has stained the integrity of the American research enterprise to a degree that will affect our thinking about research ethics and regulation for years to come. Articles and books have been written about the ethical implications of this study, and it has become a milestone in the history of research regulation. This study was the main reason that the principle of justice was developed in the Belmont Report (a topic explained in Chapter 1-4). Public reaction to the Tuskegee Study also catalyzed a series of events that led to passage of the National Research Act of 1974.

1974: THE NATIONAL RESEARCH ACT AND THE IRB SYSTEM

Following the congressional hearings directed by Senator Kennedy in 1973, the basic consensus was that federal oversight was required to protect the rights and welfare of research subjects. It is important to note that public concern was not limited to medical or biomedical research. The Wichita Jury Study, the Milgram studies, and the Tearoom Trade Study are only some of the research activities that led our congressional representatives to conclude that federal regulation should also be directed at social science research.

This chapter began by asking a key question: How did we go from almost no federal oversight of research in 1950 to the extensive system of federal laws and regulations that we have today? The short answer is that in 1974 Congress passed the National Research Act in response to a long list of events that convinced the American public that human subjects were being exploited and harmed on a regular basis by both biomedical and social science researchers. The act did two things that have had a major influence on the way research is regulated today:

1. **The National Research Act of 1974 established the modern IRB system for regulating research involving human subjects.** The act passed federal regulations that required IRB approval to conduct most kinds of research involving human subjects, defined the policy and procedures that an IRB must follow when reviewing research, and established the criteria that an IRB must use to approve research conduct. In other words, the act set up the IRB system that we use today.

   As mentioned in other sections of this handbook, it is not important for IRB members to focus on the specific regulations and federal agencies that direct IRB policy and procedures. However, some IRB members may find it useful to understand that, as directed by the National Research Act of 1974, the Department of Health and Human Services initially promulgated the main IRB regulations in 1981 in Title 45, Part 46 of the Code of Federal Regulations (45 CFR 46). These regulations were revised as recently as November 2001 and additional sections continue to be created in response to new thinking and specialized issues. In 1991 seventeen federal agencies adopted HHS regulations at 45 CFR 46. Because these regulations are now common to most federal agencies, the HHS regulations at 45 CFR 46 are referred to as the Common Rule.

While it may be confusing to those of us who are not familiar with the structure of federal agencies, IRB members may hear discussions in which a distinction is made between the Common Rule or HHS regulations and Food and Drug Administration (FDA) regulations related to IRB review of research. Again, it is not important for IRB members to understand this regulatory structure but the bottom line is that although FDA is actually part of the Department of Health and Human Services, HHS and FDA have separate regulations related to research involving human subjects. In other words, FDA has not signed on to the Common Rule. Since the differences between HHS and FDA regulations related to the IRB are minor, it will be unusual for an IRB member to be asked to understand anything about this distinction. These issues are explained in detail, and all of the relevant federal regulations reproduced, in *Institutional Review Board: Management and Function*, the textbook referenced in Chapter 1-1. HHS regulations at 45 CFR 46 (the Common Rule) are found at http://www.med. umich.edu/irbmed/FederalDocuments/hhs/HHS45 CFR46.html.

2. **The National Research Act of 1974 established the National Commission for Protection of Human Subjects of Biomedical and Behavioral Research.** The debates and hearings that led to the National Research Act of 1974 made it clear that establishing ethical standards for the conduct of research was not a simple matter. While congress did go ahead and establish specific research regulations as described above, the legislators involved with this effort recognized that there were many situations where it was difficult to know what to do. To help clarify the general guidelines that should be used to conduct research in settings that are ethically challenging, the National Research Act of 1974 created a special committee called the National Commission for Protection of Human Subjects of Biomedical and Behavioral Research. Made up of a diverse group of people representing the fields of ethics, religion, law, industry, medicine, and other disciplines, the committee is often referred to as the National Commission.

   Between 1975 and 1978 the National Commission issued multiple reports that defined problems and made recommendations regarding the conduct of research in specific populations. For example, the group published reports on research involving children, pregnant women, prisoners, and people with dementia. These population-specific reports were important in establishing the ethical framework that is used to think about research in vulnerable populations, and in many cases federal regulations and other guidelines were revised in response to the National Commission's recommendations. In 1978 the commission issued the Belmont Report, a major milestone in research ethics and research regulation. It is the subject of the next chapter.

PRINCIPLES OF THE BELMONT REPORT

ROBERT J. AMDUR

Ethical Principles of the Belmont Report

Principle 1: Respect for Persons

- Treat individuals as autonomous agents.
- Protect persons with diminished autonomy.

[Consent monitors, etc. should be considered when subjects have diminished autonomy.]

Requirements for IRB Approval
- Participants voluntarily consent to participate in research.
- Obtain informed consent
- Privacy and confidentiality are protected.

Principle 2: Beneficence

- Do unto others as you would have them do unto you.
[Trade-offs between individual and societal benefit require IRB members to make difficult choices.]

Requirements for IRB Approval
- The risks of research are justified by potential benefits to the individual or society.
- The study is designed so risks are minimized.
- Conflicts of interest are managed adequately.

Principle 3: Justice

- Distribute the risks and potential benefits of research equally among those who may benefit from the research.

Requirements for IRB Approval
- Vulnerable subjects are not targeted for convenience.
- People who are likely to benefit from research participation are not systematically excluded.

THE NATIONAL COMMISSION AND THE BELMONT REPORT

The National Research Act of 1974 established the National Commission for Protection of Human Subjects of Biomedical and Behavioral Research, a committee whose goal it was to clarify the ethical guidelines applying to research involving human subjects in any setting. After issuing a series of reports that discussed research involving especially vulnerable subject populations such as prisoners and children, the commission conducted a series of core meetings related to this work at the Belmont Conference Center near Baltimore, Maryland. The report that was issued in 1978 to explain the fundamental ethical principles that should guide the conduct of research involving human subjects became known as the Belmont Report.

The Belmont Report is an eight-page document that clearly explains the three principles that are the main tools that all IRB members should use to evaluate the ethics of specific research proposals. All IRB members should receive a copy of the Belmont Report when they are appointed to the IRB. A copy of the Belmont Report is included in *Institutional Review Board: Management and Function*, the textbook mentioned in Chapter 1-1 and it is currently online at http://ohrp.osophs.dhhs.gov/humansubjects/guidance/belmont.htm.

The remainder of this chapter will summarize the three ethical principles that are explained in the Belmont Report and explain several terms and concepts that IRB members need to understand to apply these principles when making IRB determinations.

BELMONT PRINCIPLE 1: RESPECT FOR PERSONS

The principle of respect for persons incorporates two main ethical convictions related to individual autonomy:

- Individuals are treated as autonomous agents.
- Persons with diminished autonomy are given
  protection.

There are four conditions that follow directly from this principle and are thus requirements for IRB approval of research:

- Voluntary consent to participate in research
- Informed consent to participate in research
- Protection of privacy and confidentiality
- The right to withdraw from research participation without penalty

The Right to Individual Autonomy and Self-Determination

According to the first ethical conviction involving the principle of respect for persons, each individual has the right to autonomy and self-determination. We thus give each person the right to determine his or her own destiny.

The second ethical conviction involving respect for persons involves protection of those individuals who are not capable of self-determination. Children have diminished autonomy by virtue of their intellectual development and legal status in society. Prisoners have diminished autonomy because they have forfeited certain basic personal liberties. People with certain conditions or in situations that affect their ability to think clearly have compromised autonomy when they cannot understand their situation well enough to control their own destiny. Similarly, people who do not have the educational background to understand the important implications of research participation cannot control their own destiny when they make decisions about research participation.

Vulnerable Subjects

In the language of research regulation, the term "vulnerable" is used to describe people who are likely to have compromised autonomy related to decisions about research participation to a degree that would violate the principle of respect for persons. To say that subjects are vulnerable means that they are likely to have compromised autonomy to a degree that demands extra protection.

Protecting Vulnerable Subjects

The second main ethical conviction of the principle of respect for persons is that persons with diminished autonomy are entitled to protection to prevent exploitation. In many situations it is difficult to decide if persons who are likely to have diminished autonomy should be excluded from research. Preventing people from making a decision about research participation may violate the principle of the respect for persons as it denies them the right of self-determination. When there are conflicting issues related to respect for persons, the principle itself requires judgment decisions that evaluate potential risks and benefits for specific subjects.

In addition to excluding potentially vulnerable persons from research, there are many things that researchers and/or the IRB can do specifically to increase the protection of vulnerable subjects based on diminished autonomy. For example, when subjects are incapacitated, the research plan could require informed consent from a well-educated and properly motivated surrogate decision-maker. When the potential for coercion is high, the research plan could require that an independent subject-advocate monitor the consent process. When comprehension of important information is the issue, the research plan could include provisions to test the subject's understanding of the important information prior to enrollment.

Coercion or Undue Influence Versus Voluntary Actions

In order to implement the Belmont principle—respect for persons—it is important to understand the concept of "coercion." Basically, coercion means that a person is to some degree forced, or at least strongly pushed, to do something that is not good for him or her to do. In discussions of research regulation the term "undue influence" is often used to describe the concept of coercion.

Coercion is a concept that is impossible to define beyond a certain point. Like pornography, it is difficult to define but you know it when you see it. Does your salary coerce you into going to work? If you say no, then consider whether you would quit if you didn't get paid. The point is that it is not possible to define coercion in a way that establishes a clear line between situations that are, and are not, ethical.

Coercion is unethical because individuals who are coerced into participating in research have diminished autonomy (do not have the right to control their own destiny) to the degree that the principle of respect for persons demands. Said another way, if individuals are put in a position where there is "undue influence" to participate in research, then their ability to control their own destiny has been compromised. The term that is used to explain the situation where there is no significant coercion or undue influence is "voluntary." The principle of respect for persons requires that decisions regarding research participation be made voluntarily—without coercion or undue influence.

Informed Consent

A fundamental issue for the conduct of ethical research is the concept of informed consent. According to this process, subjects must understand the important implications of the decision to participate in research, and they must actively agree to such participation. Informed consent is a condition that follows directly from the principle of respect for persons.

The conduct of research with subjects who are not competent to give informed consent is one of the most controversial issues in research ethics. Conducting research based on permission from someone other than the research subject is based on the concept of "substituted judgment" which basically means that the person making the decision knows what the subject would want to do in that situation. Obviously, such assumptions are fraught with practical and ethical problems. It is for this reason that people who are not capable of making informed decisions are described as "vulnerable" and the principle of respect for persons requires that they be given extra protection so that their right to individual autonomy is respected to an acceptable degree.

Privacy and Confidentiality

The protection of privacy and confidentiality is a concept that follows directly from the principle of respect for persons. For most IRB members, it will be useful to think of privacy and confidentiality as they relate to potentially damaging or embarrassing information about a research subject. Basically, "privacy" means that sensitive research information will not be linked to specific individuals. "Confidentiality" means that sensitive, identifiable information is collected for research purposes but access to the information is limited to a well-defined group—like the research team and the IRB.

Privacy and confidentiality are thus related to the principle of respect for persons as well as individual autonomy. Such concepts allow research subjects to control who has access to information that may harm them in any way. The harm that results from invasion of privacy or breach in confidentiality is usually called "social harm" because it compromises a person's reputation, financial status, employability, or insurability, or in some way results in stigmatization or discrimination.

BELMONT PRINCIPLE 2: BENEFICENCE

The principle of beneficence is described in the Belmont Report as being an obligation to secure the well-being of the research subject. Some people think that beneficence is just another way of emphasizing the rule of "do no harm." From the standpoint of making IRB determinations, it is probably better to think of this principle as a commitment that goes beyond "do no harm" to include the conviction that research should be designed to maximize potential benefits and minimize potential risks.

Most IRB members will find it useful to translate the term "beneficence" into something more familiar that captures the important aspects of this fundamental ethical principle. Some experienced IRB members prefer to think of beneficence as a requirement to "be kind to subjects" or to "do unto others as you would have them do unto you." IRB members should use these standards when evaluating research proposals. Specifically:

- To determine if a research proposal supports the principle of beneficence each IRB member should ask the following question: "Are research subjects treated the way that I would like to be treated in this situation?"

The principle of beneficence also requires IRB members to evaluate the risks and potential benefits of research participation:

- The risks of research are justified by the potential benefits to the individual and/or society.

Note: The IRB is often forced to make a value judgment about the trade-off between the implications of research for the individual versus those of society. The Belmont Report acknowledges that this is an unavoidable conflict that must be resolved on a case-by-case basis.

- The study is designed so that risks are minimized and potential benefits are maximized.

Note: This means that the IRB is required to evaluate the quality of the science in a research proposal, the qualifications of the investigator, the resources available to accomplish the study as planned, and the methods used in the study relative to the available alternatives. It is the principle of beneficence that directs the IRB to evaluate fundamental aspects of study design such as the characteristics of the control group and the statistical power calculations.

• Conflicts of interest are managed so that bias in important judgments related to research conduct is unlikely.

Note: A conflict of interest that is likely to bias important judgments about the conduct of research violates the principle of beneficence because it means that risks to subjects are not minimized.

BELMONT PRINCIPLE 3: JUSTICE

The principle of justice is more difficult to understand and implement than the principles of respect for persons and beneficence because the concept of justice relates to the distribution of risk within society. It may be useful to understand that the Belmont Report defined the principle of justice in response to studies that appeared to exploit some of the most vulnerable segments of our society (see Chapter 1-3). As explained in the Belmont Report, the principle of justice basically says the following:

• The potential risks of research should be born equally by the members of our society that are likely to benefit from it.

Note: To apply the principle of justice when evaluating a research proposal, the IRB must evaluate the characteristics of the study population:

• The research project does not systematically select specific classes or types of individuals simply because of their ease of availability or their compromised position as opposed to reasons directly related to the problem being studied.

Note: The Belmont report mentions welfare patients, particular racial or ethnic minorities, and persons confined to institutions as examples of classes of subjects that would raise concern based on the principle of justice.

The above discussion summarizes the principle of justice as it is described in the Belmont Report. The traditional application of the principle of justice has focused on which subjects are *included* in research when they should not be. However, in the past twenty years the principle of justice has been reinterpreted to mean that it is unethical to *exclude* classes of people who are likely to benefit from research participation or in whom the results of a specific kind of research are likely to be applied. Specific examples of this interpretation of the principle of justice are the exclusion of women of childbearing potential from Phase 3 investigational drug trials and the exclusion of children from research involving investigational drugs that are primarily used in adults. Both practices are currently being challenged on the grounds that it violates the principle of justice to deny these groups the benefit of knowing how research results apply to them. If one accepts this interpretation of the principle of justice, the principle of justice also requires the following:

• The research project does not systematically exclude a specific class or type of person who is likely to benefit from research participation or in whom the results of a specific kind of research are likely to be applied.

PART 2

The Full-Committee IRB Meeting

CHAPTER 2-1

THE WORK BEFORE AN IRB MEETING

ROBERT J. AMDUR AND LIZ BANKERT

Do the Work of IRB Review Before the Meeting

- Review your assigned information at least two days before the meeting.
- Consider the IRB meeting to be primarily a place to make decisions, not gather information.
- Get your questions answered before the IRB meeting.
- Discuss your assignments with the investigator, other IRB members, or consultants prior to the IRB meeting.
- Do not hesitate to discuss the protocol with the investigator.
- Before the meeting, inform the IRB chair and/or other members if you have concerns about a proposal.
- Decide if the investigator should attend the meeting.
- If you want the investigator to make specific changes in the language of the application or consent document, come to the meeting with the application rewritten so that it reads the way that you want it to.

The purpose of this chapter is to emphasize the importance of doing the majority of the work of IRB review before the full-committee IRB meeting. Identifying and evaluating ethical issues are often time-consuming and complex processes. To be an effective IRB member, you have to be willing and able to conduct a thorough review of research proposals prior to the IRB meeting. The guidelines presented in this chapter apply to all types of agenda items—initial protocol review, revisions, and continuing reviews. For IRBs that use a primary reviewer system, these guidelines apply most directly to the IRB members that are assigned to a specific agenda item. The bottom line is clear: If you want to have a major impact on the protection of research subjects, you have to follow the golden rule of IRB review:

- Do most of the work of IRB review <u>BEFORE</u> the meeting.

The guidelines listed below are specific behaviors that follow directly from the golden rule.

- Review your assigned information at least two days before the meeting.

The IRB will not function optimally if members wait until the night before the meeting to review their assignments. Ideally, all IRB members will receive the paperwork they need at least a week before the meeting. At an absolute minimum, members should have two full days to work on their assignments.

- Consider the IRB meeting to be primarily a place to make decisions, not gather information.

An effective IRB will use the full-committee meeting time to debate issues and make the difficult determinations that are required to meaningfully influence the protection of research subjects. It is counterproductive to use the meeting time for things that could have been done more effectively before the meeting.

- Get your questions answered *before* the IRB meeting.

A thorough IRB review usually means that you will need clarification or additional information about aspects of a research proposal. The IRB meeting is not the best place for most of these activities. Ideally, the IRB chair will establish clear expectations for each IRB member. Review your assignments ahead of time and come to the meeting with the information you need to make an informed recommendation about how the committee should vote on the issue.

• Discuss your assignments with the investigator, other IRB members, or consultants prior to the IRB meeting.

This is especially true for new protocol reviews but also applies to other types of assignments when the information presented is complex or troublesome. IRB members are not expected to be absolute experts in the proposals that they review. Even when IRB members are knowledgeable about the type of research that they are reviewing, interaction with other people will be required to make informed determinations.

• Do not hesitate to discuss the protocol with the investigator.

Collegial interaction between investigators and IRB reviewers will facilitate the IRB review process and promote respect for the local IRB system. The IRB chair or administrative director should encourage members to directly contact investigators for further information or clarification. However, the IRB office should serve as an intermediary for any IRB member who may wish to obtain further information but does not have time to (or prefers not to) personally follow up with the investigator. Investigators who resist talking with IRB reviewers or criticize them for requesting clarification or justification of important ethical issues demonstrate a lack of respect for the system of protecting research subjects that has been mandated by the organization for which the IRB serves. A lack of respect in this setting is an important finding that should be taken into account when making IRB determinations.

- Before the meeting, inform the IRB chair and/or
  other IRB members if you have concerns about a
  proposal.

The key message of this chapter is that IRB reviewers
should make every attempt to resolve issues of concern
prior to the meeting. This is not to suggest that there will
not be issues that need to be discussed or debated at the
full committee meeting. An IRB that does not routinely
struggle with controversial or potentially troublesome
issues is probably not doing a good job.

When IRB members have issues that they are not able to
resolve prior to a meeting, they should be sure that the
IRB chair and/or other assigned reviewers are informed
about the issues that are of concern or need specific clar-
ifications. This gives IRB members the time they need to
prepare for a knowledgeable discussion at the meeting.
Electronic mail is an efficient way to give everyone a
"heads up" about issues of concern before the meeting.

- Decide if the investigator should attend the meeting.

Some IRBs require an investigator to attend the IRB
meeting whenever a new protocol is being reviewed.
Most IRBs find that it is not productive to require the
investigator to attend the IRB meeting on a regular basis.
When there is a question about whether the principal
investigator or other important members of the research
team will be present at the IRB meeting, it is important
for the primary reviewers to decide if the investigator's
presence at the meeting will facilitate IRB review of the
protocol. When reviewers think that it will be useful for
an investigator to attend the meeting, they should ask the
IRB administrator to inform the investigator of this with
as much lead time as possible.

The most common reason that the IRB should ask an
investigator to attend the IRB meeting is to discuss an
important issue that could not be resolved before the
meeting. Another good reason might involve a situation

where the reviewer thinks it will be important for other IRB members to hear an investigator explain something personally rather than to have the reviewer explain to the committee that there is no reason to be concerned. When an investigator is asked to attend the IRB meeting, the primary reviewer should give the investigator as clear an idea as possible why his or her presence at the meeting may be useful. ₀

• If you want the investigator to make specific changes in the language of the application or consent document, come to the meeting with the application rewritten so that it reads the way that you want it to.

Doing the work of the IRB review before the meeting means that you identify the changes in the application, consent document, or protocol that you think should be a requirement for IRB approval. Respect for the IRB process is compromised when an IRB tables a proposal because the committee wants the investigator to change the way he or she answered a certain question on the IRB submission form or worded the research protocol. The consent document is discussed in more detail in Chapter 2-3. The bottom line is that the IRB meeting is certainly not the place to spend time polishing the wording of the consent document. In most cases wording or response changes should be discussed, and resolved, with the investigator before the meeting. In cases where it is not possible to have the necessary revisions made prior to the meeting, the IRB reviewers should come to the meeting with an explicit recommendation for how the proposal should be revised.

REVIEWING A NEW RESEARCH PROPOSAL

ROBERT J. AMDUR, SUSAN KORNETSKY, AND
LIZ BANKERT

Using a Systematic Approach to Review a New Protocol Application

- Establish a routine for reviewing the application package:

  1. Read the consent document but don't take notes or make revisions.

  2. Read the protocol summary.

  3. Read the full protocol and supporting material carefully. Take notes as needed.

  4. Reread the consent document.

- Use a reviewer template, such as the one shown in this chapter.

Scenario: You have been assigned to be a primary reviewer for a new protocol and have just sat down to review the IRB application package a few days before the full-committee meeting. You are looking at a thick stack of papers that include things like an application checklist, a summary of the protocol, a detailed description of protocol procedures, and a consent document. You have to decide what to read first and how to structure your review. The purpose of this chapter is to suggest an approach that will make the process of your review more effective and more efficient.

USING A SYSTEMATIC APPROACH TO REVIEW THE APPLICATION MATERIAL

It is important to develop a formal system for reviewing the application material. What works well for one reviewer, however, may not be the best system for another. Use the approach that works best for you. Some experienced IRB reviewers favor the following:

1. **Read the consent document:** Because the purpose of the consent document is to explain the important aspects of the study to potential subjects in lay language, it should give you a good introduction to the protocol. During this initial reading, you should not take notes or attempt to correct the wording of the document. The purpose of this reading is to orient yourself with the overall design of the study.

2. **Read the protocol summary:** After completing an overview of the study based on the consent form, review the summary of the protocol submitted as part of the IRB application. The IRB summary protocol is the part of the application where the investigator summarizes the important aspects of the study in a way that facilitates IRB review.

3. **Read the full protocol and supporting material:** Read the supporting material that completes the information presented in the IRB application form. For example, primary reviewers receive the full sponsor protocol from the study sponsor. This will provide the reviewer with detailed information such as prior studies that are applicable to the study treatment or that validate study procedures, statistical power analysis, detailed inclusion/exclusion requirements, and recruitment advertisements.

4. **Read the consent document again:** This time, record suggested corrections or questions for the investigator.

USING A REVIEWER TEMPLATE

A reviewer template is a form that lists the main issues or questions that an IRB reviewer evaluates when reviewing a new protocol. Such a template will help you organize the review and remember what issues have and have not been addressed. It is also useful for presenting the review at the full committee meeting, and it can be kept in the IRB file as documentation that a detailed review was performed. Many reviewers create their own templates according to the format that works best for them, but some IRB offices ask every reviewer to use the same template, which in certain cases may be lengthy and extremely detailed. In our opinion, the primary purpose of the reviewer template is to help the reviewer evaluate the protocol and explain it to other IRB members. For this reason, it is useful to keep the template as short and simple as possible. A sample one-page template is included below. The most applicable Belmont Report principle is shown in boldface after each item to remind the reviewer why the information is important.

IRB Primary Reviewer Template   Study No.:_____

(Write on the other side of this page as needed.)

Reviewer:_____ Date:_____

Purpose of study:

Summary (Background, number of arms, controls, IND, etc.)

Sponsor

Investigator (Qualified? Conflict of interest?) [Beneficence]

Study population and recruitment practices
Includes vulnerable subjects (Children, etc.)? [Respect for Persons]
Subject recruitment (Who, where, how?) [Beneficence]
Payment or reimbursements (Coercive?) [Beneficence]
Is subject selection likely to be equitable? [Justice]
Adequacy of procedures to protect vulnerable subjects [Respect for Persons]

Informed consent (Written, surrogate, etc.) [Respect for Persons]

Birth control [Beneficence]

Genetic testing/tissue repository [Respect for Persons and Beneficence]
Will the subjects or their doctors be given research results? Are they informed of this before enrolling?
Cost (relative to nonresearch cost)
Will subjects understand increased cost? [Respect for Persons]
Are subjects coerced to accept increased cost? [Beneficence]

Risks (relative to nonresearch alternative) [Beneficence]
Rate risk level as (1) minimal, (2) moderate, or (3) high:
Absolute _____ Relative _____
Risks are minimized. (Appropriate control group?)

Potential benefit (Direct for the subject versus altruism)

Risk/benefit analysis [Beneficence]
Risks are minimized and reasonable in view of potential benefits.

Confidentiality [Respect for Persons]
Provisions to protect privacy and confidentiality are adequate.

Data oversight [Beneficence]
How will data be monitored?
Stopping rules are explained and sufficiently detailed.

Consent document [Respect for Persons]
Accurately describes the essential elements in a way that is likely to be understood by the expected subject population:

A MORE DETAILED REVIEWER WORKSHEET

A reviewer worksheet is a tool that assists IRB members in reviewing research protocols. In some institutions, use of a worksheet is suggested; in others, the worksheet is mandatory. This section presents a version of the worksheet that is used at Children's Hospital in Boston, Massachusetts. All of the information related to this worksheet is taken from a chapter written by Susan Kornetsky in *Institutional Review Board: Management and Function*, the textbook recommended in Chapter 1-1.

The worksheet is divided into eleven sections; each addresses one of the criteria for IRB approval as specified in the regulations and presents specific questions and criteria to be considered. In addition, in some sections members can write questions or concerns that an investigator needs to address. The worksheet sections thus prompt IRB members to make specific determinations for an individual protocol.

INTRODUCTION, SPECIFIC AIMS, AND BACKGROUND

- Are the specific aims clearly specified?
- Are there adequate preliminary data to justify the research?
- Is there appropriate justification for this research protocol?

SCIENTIFIC DESIGN

- Is the scientific design adequate to answer the question?
- Are the objectives likely to be achievable within a given time period?
- Is the scientific design (i.e., randomization; placebo controls; Phase 1, 2, or 3) described and adequately justified?

INCLUSION/EXCLUSION CRITERIA FOR SUBJECTS

- Are inclusion and exclusion criteria clearly specified and appropriate?
- If women, minorities, or children are included or excluded, is this justified?
- Is the choice of subjects appropriate for the question being asked?
- Is the principle of distributive justice adequately incorporated into the inclusion and exclusion criteria for the research protocol? Is subject selection equitable?

RECRUITMENT OF SUBJECTS

- Are the methods for recruiting potential subjects well defined?
- Are the location and timing of the recruitment process acceptable?
- Is the individual performing the recruitment appropriate for the process?
- Are all recruitment materials submitted and appropriate?
- Are there acceptable methods for screening subjects before recruitment?

RESEARCH PROCEDURES

- Are the rationale and details of the research procedures accurately described and acceptable?
- Is there a clear differentiation between research procedures and standard care?
- Are the individuals performing the procedures appropriately trained, and is the location of performing the procedure acceptable?
- Are there adequate plans to inform subjects about specific research results if necessary (clinically relevant results, risk of depression, suicidality, incidental findings, etc.)?

DRUGS, BIOLOGICS, AND DEVICES

- Is the status of the drug described and appropriate (investigational, new use of an FDA-approved drug, or an FDA-approved drug within approved indications)?
- Are the drug dosage and route of administration appropriate?
- Are the drug or device safety and efficacy data sufficient to warrant the proposed phase of testing?
- Is the significant risk or nonsignificant risk status of the device described and appropriate?

DATA ANALYSIS AND STATISTICAL ANALYSIS

- Is the rationale for the proposed number of subjects reasonable?
- Are the plans for data and statistical analysis defined and justified, including the use of stopping rules and endpoints?
- Are there adequate provisions for monitoring data (DSMB)?

POTENTIAL RISKS, DISCOMFORTS, AND BENEFITS FOR SUBJECTS

- Are the risks and benefits adequately identified, evaluated, and described?
- Are the potential risks minimized and likelihood of benefits maximized?
- Is the risk/benefit ratio acceptable for proceeding with the research?
- If children are involved, which regulatory category of risk/benefit does the protocol fall within and are all criteria within the category adequately addressed?

COMPENSATION AND COSTS FOR SUBJECTS

- Is the amount or type of compensation or reimbursement reasonable?

- Are there adequate provisions to avoid out-of-pocket expenses by the research subject, or is there sufficient justification to allow subjects to pay?

- If children or adolescents are involved, who receives the compensation, and is this appropriate?

PRIVACY AND CONFIDENTIALITY

- Are there adequate provisions to protect the privacy and ensure the confidentiality of the research subject?

- Are there adequate plans to store and code the data?

- Is the use of identifiers or links to identifiers necessary, and how is this information protected?

OTHER ISSUES

- Are adequate references provided?

- When should the next review occur? If frequent reviews are necessary, how should the interval be determined?

THE CONSENT DOCUMENT

ROBERT J. AMDUR AND LIZ BANKERT

Guidelines for Reviewing the Consent Document

The following information must be included in the consent document per federal regulations:

- Research purpose and procedures
- Risks and discomforts
- Potential benefits
- Alternative procedures or treatment
- Provisions for confidentiality
- Research-related injury
- Contacts for additional information
- Voluntary participation and the right to discontinue participation without penalty

When appropriate, the consent document should describe the following additional information:

- Unforeseeable risks
- Termination of participation by the investigator
- Additional costs
- Consequences of discontinuing research participation
- Notification of significant new findings
- Approximate number of subjects

The key message of this chapter is that revision of the consent document should be a small part of the review process. Most IRB members and committees spend too much time polishing the wording of the consent document. After the consent document explains the important implications of a decision to participate in research, the wording of the consent document does little to protect the rights and welfare of research participants. Most subjects get the information that they need to make an informed decision by discussing the protocol with members of the research team as well as with family and friends. This is especially true in the current research environment where IRBs routinely approve consent documents that are lengthy and complex.

Here are the guidelines that IRB members should follow when reviewing the consent document:

- **Use the term "consent document" or "consent form" instead of "informed consent":** Informed consent is an action—an ongoing process of communication between the subject and research staff. Informed consent is not a document, and presenting subjects with information in a document does not constitute informed consent.

- **Resist the urge to make unimportant changes to the consent document:** Although things may not be explained as clearly as they could be, once the consent document presents the main implications of research participation, polishing the wording of the document will not meaningfully improve the protection of research subjects. When considering a change in the consent document, ask yourself "Is this change likely to have an important impact on the protection of research subjects?" If the answer is no, don't make the change.

- **If you want to revise the consent document, record your changes in writing before the IRB meeting:** Doing the work of IRB review prior to the meeting is the message of Chapter 2-1.

- **If you want to make substantive changes, such as adding major risks or eliminating potential benefits, make an effort to discuss the changes with the investigator before the meeting:** It is important to identify issues of contention before the meeting so that all parties can explain their view before the IRB makes a determination.

- **The consent document should be written in lay language:** Although it is difficult to define what is meant by "lay language," the point is that the consent document should be written so that the intended subject population is likely to understand the important information. There is much talk about requiring the consent document to be written at the eighth- or tenth-grade level, and there are word processing programs that profess to evaluate this. Most IRBs find these programs of little value because the concepts are artificial. There is no substitute for having someone read the consent document and make subjective decisions about the complexity of the language.

- **The primary reviewer must determine that the consent document contains the information required by federal regulations:** Federal regulations list eight essential elements of informed consent that must be described in the consent document, and the regulations require that additional information be explained in certain circumstances. Since the first required element has four subsections there are actually thirteen items that the consent document should contain. The information that the consent document should contain is presented below in the format used by the federal regulations:

Information That Must Be Included in the Consent Document per Federal Regulations

1. **Research purpose and procedures:** a statement that the study involves research, an explanation of the purposes of the research and the expected duration of the subject's participation, a description of the procedures to be followed, and identification of any procedures which are experimental;

2. **Risks and discomforts:** a description of any reasonably foreseeable risks or discomforts to the subject;

3. **Potential benefits:** a description of any benefits to the subject or to others that may reasonably be expected from the research;

4. **Alternative procedures or treatments:** a disclosure of appropriate alternative procedures or courses of treatment, if any, that might be advantageous to the subject;

5. **Provisions for confidentiality:** a statement describing the extent, if any, to which confidentiality of records identifying the subject will be maintained;

6. **Research-related injury:** for research involving more than minimal risk, an explanation as to whether any compensation and any medical treatments are available if injury occurs and, if so, what they consist of, or where further information may be obtained;

7. **Contacts for additional information:** an explanation of whom to contact for answers to pertinent questions about the research and research subject's rights, and whom to contact in the event of a research-related injury to the subject; and

8. **Voluntary participation and the right to discontinue participation without penalty:** a statement that participation is voluntary, refusal to participate will involve no penalty or loss of benefits to which the subject is otherwise entitled, and the subject may discontinue participation at any time without penalty or loss of benefits to which the subject is otherwise entitled.

When appropriate, the consent document should include the following additional information:

9. **Unforeseeable risks:** a statement that the particular treatment or procedure may involve risks to the subject (or to the embryo or fetus, if the subject is or may become pregnant) which are currently unforeseeable;

10. **Termination of participation by the investigator:** anticipated circumstances under which the subject's participation may be terminated by the investigator without regard to the subject's consent;

11. **Additional costs:** any additional costs to the subject that may result from participation in the research;

12. **Consequences of discontinuing research participation:** the consequences of a subject's decision to withdraw from the research and procedures for orderly termination of participation by the subject;

13. **Notification of significant new findings:** a statement that significant new findings developed during the course of the research that may relate to the subject's willingness to continue participation will be provided to the subject; and

14. **Approximate number of subjects:** the approximate number of subjects involved in the study.

CONTINUING REVIEW OF RESEARCH

ROBERT J. AMDUR AND LIZ BANKERT

Guidelines for Continuing Review of Research

- Determine if the study is currently actively enrolling, treating, or following subjects.
- Determine that the number of subjects enrolled at the IRB's institution does not exceed the number that the study was initially approved for.
- Review any requested protocol revisions and any protocol revisions that have been approved by the IRB since the last continuing review.
- Determine if the study is progressing as planned.
- Determine if unexpected events have occurred that may indicate a need for a change in the protocol or consent.
- Determine if information has become available since starting the study that indicates a need to make modifications.
- Determine if subjects have registered any grievances or complaints about this study.
- Determine whether the consent document that is currently in use contains all previous revisions
- Review a current report from the data monitoring mechanism to determine that study events are being evaluated relative to the appropriate stopping or modification rules.

A continuing review of research begins as soon as a study is initiated. The usual mechanism for such a review is an Adverse Event Report or an interim report on the project to the IRB. Most studies undergo annual IRB review, but in situations of increased risk continuing review should be required more frequently. A review can be handled according to the primary reviewer system, as is done with initial protocol review. The guidelines for continuing IRB review of previously approved protocols are presented below. It is useful for the IRB to develop a standardized form that leads the investigator and reviewer through the important issues:

- Verify that all of the criteria for approval of research at the time of initial review apply to IRB approval of research at the time of continuing review. IRB members should review the criteria discussed in Chapter 2-2 when conducting a continuing review of protocols.
- Determine the current status of the study. There are several options:

  - Active
  - Closed to enrollment, and participants continue to receive study treatment
  - Closed to enrollment, and subjects are not receiving study treatment but follow-up procedures are different from what would be done off-protocol
  - Closed to enrollment subjects are not receiving study treatment, and follow-up procedures are identical to what would be done off-protocol

- Determine that the number of subjects enrolled at the IRB's institution does not exceed, and is not likely to exceed in the near future, the number that the study was initially approved for.
- Review any protocol revisions that have been approved by the IRB since the last continuing review.
- Review any requested protocol revisions that have not been previously approved by the IRB.
- Determine if the study is progressing as planned. It is useful to ask the investigator an open-ended question about the progress of the study as planned.
- Determine if unexpected events, toxicity, or complications have occurred that may indicate a need for a change in the protocol or consent. This is another way of saying that an important focus of the contin-

uing review is to determine if the risk/benefit profile has changed since the initial protocol application was reviewed. It is useful to ask the investigator to address this question.

- Determine if information (publications, presentations, etc.) has become available since starting the study that indicates a need to make modifications. This is also a question about changes in the risk/benefit profile. Again, it is useful to ask the investigator to address this question.
- Determine if subjects have registered any grievances or complaints about this study. Again, it is useful to ask the investigator to address this question.
- Determine whether the consent document that is currently in use contains all previous revisions.
- Review a current report from the data-monitoring mechanism (Principal Investigator, Data-Monitoring Committee, or Data Safety Monitoring Board) to determine that study events are being evaluated relative to the appropriate stopping or modification rules. A detailed description of the plan for data monitoring throughout the course of the study should be a requirement for IRB approval at the time of initial protocol review. This includes the person or group that will be responsible for reviewing this information, the frequency of data analysis, the endpoints that will be evaluated, the criteria that will be used to stop or modify the study, and the timing of reports to the IRB. At the time of continuing review, the IRB should require documentation that data monitoring is being conducted as planned. It is appropriate for the IRB to require a protocol revision to improve the plans for data monitoring if the IRB thinks this will improve the protection of research subjects.

PROTOCOL REVISIONS (AMENDMENTS)

ROBERT J. AMDUR AND LIZ BANKERT

Guidelines for Review of Protocol Revisions (Amendments)

1. Identify the part of the research proposal that is being revised:

   - Administrative details (research personnel, phone numbers, etc.)
   - Inclusion or exclusion criteria
   - Testing frequency or methods (a new questionnaire, more frequent blood draws, etc.)
   - Treatment parameters
   - Stopping or modification rules
   - Consent document
   - Recruitment procedures (payment schedules, advertisements, etc.)

2. Determine if the revision increases risk for *currently enrolled* subjects.

3. Determine if the revision increases risk for *future* subjects.

4. Determine if the consent document should be revised or if the proposed revision to the consent document is adequate.

5. Determine if currently enrolled subjects should be reconsented.

6. If the proposed revision increases risk to current or future subjects, determine if the protocol still meets the criteria that are used to evaluate new studies (Chapter 2-2).

The term "amendment" is often used to describe additions or changes to the research protocol or consent document. "Protocol revision" is another term commonly used. It refers to any changes to the information that was previously approved by the IRB. Federal regulations require that all revisions be approved by the IRB prior to their implementation. While the regulations permit an IRB to approve minimal risk revisions with an expedited process, many IRBs elect to review all revisions at the full-committee meeting. Revisions that increase the risk of research participation must be approved by the full IRB committee. It is for this reason that IRB members will be assigned to review protocol revisions as separate agenda items at the full-committee meeting. The criteria for approving a protocol revision are the same as those described in Chapter 2-2 for approval of a new research proposal. Similarly, any proposed revision to the consent document must meet the requirements for such documents discussed in Chapter 2-3. However, in most cases the review of a proposed revision can be more focused than the process of initial protocol review. The important issues to consider are presented below. Most IRBs use a separate form to guide the review of proposed revisions.

1. What general part of the research proposal is being revised?

   - Administrative details (research personnel, phone numbers, etc.)
   - Inclusion or exclusion criteria
   - Testing frequency or methods (a new questionnaire, more frequent blood draws, etc.)
   - Treatment parameters
   - Stopping or modification rules
   - Consent document
   - Recruitment procedures (payment schedules, advertisements, etc.)

Other:

2. Does the revision increase risk for *currently enrolled* subjects?

   • The revision does not increase risk.
   • The risk of the revision is minimal.
   • The risk of the revision is more than minimal.

3. Does the revision increase risk for future subjects?

   • The revision does not increase risk.
   • The risk of the revision is minimal.
   • The risk of the revision is more than minimal.

4. If the revision is not to the consent document, should the consent document be revised as well?

5. Should currently enrolled subjects be reconsented, and, if so, are there provisions to do so?

6. If the proposed revision increases risk to current or future subjects, does the protocol still meet the criteria that are used to evaluate new studies? (See Chapter 2-2.)

ADVERSE EVENT REPORTS

ROBERT J. AMDUR AND LIZ BANKERT

IRB Review of Adverse Event Reports

- Is the event being reported both serious *and* unexpected?   Yes __ No__

- The IRB is required to review only events that are both serious and unexpected.

- Does a determination of the implication of this adverse event for the risk/benefit profile of research participation require a comparison of the observed and expected frequency of this event in the study population?

  If your answer to this question is Yes, answer the next question:

- Is the observed to expected comparison being evaluated at the appropriate intervals by a person or group that is qualified to make these comparisons in a time frame that will protect the welfare of research participants?

- Does this adverse event suggest that there is a meaningful change in the risk/benefit profile of research participation?

  If this adverse event does suggest that the risk/benefit profile of research participation has changed, a determination about the need to revise the study protocol and/or the consent document must be made:

- Is a revision in the study protocol required to minimize the risk of research participation?

- Should the document be revised to discuss the adverse event?

- Should currently enrolled subjects be reconsented?

- Should the frequency or nature of IRB continuing review of this protocol be changed to monitor the study more closely as a result of this adverse event?

The role of the IRB in reviewing adverse event reports is one of the most ill-defined topics in the field of research regulation, and guidance from federal authorities has been both confusing and contradictory. Countless journal articles and chapters in books have been written on this subject, but at present there is no consensus within the regulatory community about the definition of an adverse event and related issues: when the IRB should review an adverse event that occurred at an outside institution, the approach the IRB should use to evaluate an adverse event report, and the criteria an IRB should use for requiring a revision in the research plan or consent document based on an adverse event report. In view of these uncertainties, it is not surprising that IRB members are often frustrated when they review adverse event reports at the full-committee meeting or as part of an expedited-review process.

It is beyond the scope of this book to discuss the adverse event issue in detail. A thorough review of the subject is presented in *Institutional Review Board: Management and Function*, the textbook recommended in Chapter 1-1. The purpose of this chapter is to suggest a framework for reviewing adverse event reports that is easy to incorporate into a one-page review form. It has worked well for several experienced IRBs and, in our opinion, satisfies the requirements of federal regulations.

• Use a specialized form to guide the review of an
  adverse event report.

As with other kinds of IRB review, a specialized form for reviewing adverse event reports helps reviewers remember the issues that they should consider, improves the efficiency of the review process, and provides the necessary documentation for the IRB record. Each IRB should develop a form that fits best with the type of research they review and the philosophy of their institution regarding the role of the IRB in this setting. We favor a single-page form that places much of the responsibility for evaluating the significance of the adverse event on the principal investigator, and it reflects the philosophy that the role of the IRB is to confirm that an effective data monitoring mechanism is in place but that the IRB should usually not be that mechanism. The IRB should not attempt to function as a Data-Monitoring Committee or Data Safety Monitoring Board. The subsequent sections of this chapter describe the information that the IRB should evaluate when reviewing an adverse event report. Each section contains the question or statement that would be used in the one-page Adverse Event Report Review Form that will help IRBs review adverse event reports in a detailed and consistent manner. We recommend that the IRB require the principal investigator to answer each of the questions needed to evaluate an adverse event report prior to IRB review.

• Is the event being reported serious and unexpected?
  Yes __ No __

  Serious: Death, a life-threatening experience, inpatient hospitalization or prolongation of existing hospitalization, a persistent or significant disability/incapacity, or a congenital anomaly/birth defect.

  Unexpected: Any adverse experience the specificity or severity of which is not consistent with the current protocol description that was approved by the IRB or the currently approved consent form.

If the answer to this question is "Yes" (the event is serious and unexpected), the investigator and/or IRB reviewer should answer the questions below. If the answer is "No," our interpretation of federal regulations is that the IRB is not required to review the event and such review will not meaningfully improve the protection of research subjects. Many research sponsors and principal investigators are confused about this point and will request that the IRB review events that are either not serious, not unexpected, or both. In our opinion the IRB does not have time to do things that do not meaningfully contribute to the protection of research subjects. For this reason we recommend that IRBs refuse to review adverse events that are not both serious and unexpected.

- Is the adverse event currently discussed in the consent document or protocol summary (investigator brochure)? Yes ___ No ___
- If the adverse event is discussed in the version of the consent or protocol summary that was previously approved by the IRB, indicate where the event is currently discussed: Consent document _____
  Protocol summary _____

In view of the confusion about the guidelines for adverse event reporting, it is not unusual to see events come before the IRB that were anticipated in this study population. While it is our opinion that such events need not be reviewed by the IRB because they are not "unanticipated," some duplication in the review form is useful to clarify the important issues. An event that is described in the consent document or protocol summary was clearly anticipated prior to starting the study. The event may be unanticipated in frequency, but it is not unexpected to observe the event in some of the study subjects.

Another reason to determine if the adverse event is currently described in the consent document is that IRB review of an adverse event report should include a decision about revising the consent document and reconsenting enrolled subjects. These issues are addressed in separate questions below.

- How would you classify this event:
  serious but not fatal ___ fatal ___

- Briefly describe the adverse event: _____
  _____
  _____

- Where did the adverse event occur?
  local institution ___ outside institution ___

The "local" versus "outside" distinction is important in multisite studies. A local adverse event is an event that occurred in an institution that the relevant IRB is directly responsible for. An outside event is one that occurred at an institution that the IRB is not responsible for.

• Was the adverse event related to participation in this research study? Not related ___ Unlikely ___ Possibly ___ Probably ___ Definitely related ___

We include this question because many discussions of this subject in the literature make an important distinction between those events that are, versus those that are not, related to research participation. While this certainly is an important issue, the point of adverse event monitoring is to review events that could change the risk of research participation. Therefore, from the standpoint of research regulation or research ethics, the term "adverse event" refers only to events that are, or could be, caused by research participation. Events that are clearly not related to research participation should not be reported to the IRB or discussed in the context of research regulation because they have no impact on the ethics of research conduct.

OBSERVED VERSUS EXPECTED FREQUENCY COMPARISON

• Does a determination of the implication of this adverse event for the risk/benefit profile of research participation require a comparison of the observed and expected frequency of this event in the study population? Yes ___ No ___

If your answer to this question is "Yes" answer the next question.

• Is the observed to expected comparison being evaluated at the appropriate intervals by a person or group that is qualified to make the comparisons in a time frame that will protect the welfare of research participants? Yes __ No __

If your answer to this question is "Yes" answer the next question.

• Who is making the comparisons required to appropriately evaluate this adverse event:
  Principal investigator ____
  Data monitoring committee ____
  Independent data safety monitoring board ____

The concept that many events can only be interpreted by calculating observed and expected frequency rates is difficult for some people to understand, and many IRBs and investigators are not used to thinking in these terms. However, it is essential that IRB members understand the limitations of IRB review of individual adverse event reports. In most settings, the main risk of research participation is not that a totally unknown toxicity will occur but rather that an expected toxicity or adverse outcome will occur at a higher than expected frequency.

For example, consider a trial that involves a randomized comparison of best standard therapy plus or minus an investigational drug designed to improve survival following a heart attack. A major risk of study participation is that the study drug will do something harmful that leads to decreased survival. However, most IRBs have no way to evaluate the issue of increased mortality from individual adverse event reports. The IRB will usually not have "the denominator" needed to make frequency calculations, the resources available to perform the necessary statistical comparisons, or the expertise available to make observed versus expected comparisons in a given study population. There is no way for the IRB to get this information, and the IRB should not attempt to do so.

Federal regulations require the IRB to determine that the research plan provides for the monitoring of data in a way that will protect the welfare of research participants, but multiple federal guidance documents clearly explain that the IRB is not expected to be that mechanism with many types of studies. At the time of initial protocol review, the IRB is suppose to determine if the principal investigator, a Data-Monitoring Committee, or an independent Data Safety Monitoring Board will monitor data in an ongoing manner from the standpoint of subject safety and that the details of the monitoring process are appropriate. In multicenter trials, or in any trial where the study populations are large, meaningful IRB review of an adverse event report requires that the IRB determine that someone other than the IRB is monitoring the event as planned.

CHANGE IN THE RISK/BENEFIT PROFILE

• Does this adverse event suggest that there is a meaningful change in the risk/benefit profile of research participation for subjects who are currently enrolled in the study? Yes __ No __

  Briefly explain how the risk/benefit profile may change: _____
  _____
  _____

• If this adverse event does suggest that the risk/benefit profile of research participation has changed, should the study protocol (the methods, inclusion/exclusion criteria, etc.) be revised to minimize the risk of research participation (including the option of study suspension or closure)? Yes __ No __

If this adverse event does suggest that the risk/benefit profile of research participation has changed, a determination about the need to revise the study protocol and/or the consent document must be made.

• Is a revision in the study protocol required to minimize the risk of research participation?
  Yes __ No __

- Should the document be revised to discuss the adverse event? Yes ___ No ___

- Should currently enrolled subjects be reconsented? Yes ___ No ___

- Should the frequency or nature of IRB continuing review of this protocol be changed to monitor the study more closely as a result of this adverse event? Yes ___ No ___

PRIMARY REVIEWER PRESENTATIONS

ROBERT J. AMDUR AND LIZ BANKERT

Primary Reviewer Presentations at the Full-Committee Meeting

- Limit the initial summary of your review to one to two minutes.

- Your presentation should consist of reading your review form.

- Resist the urge to impress the committee with how much work you did.

- Presentations by secondary reviewers should focus on areas of disagreement with previous reviewers.

- Do not allow questions until after all of the primary reviewers have made their presentations.

- End your presentation with a vote recommendation.

In order for an IRB to function optimally, it is important that IRB members use an organized format for presenting their reviews at a full-committee meeting. The importance of using a review form to guide and document the review process was discussed in previous chapters. Each type of IRB review (new protocols, continuing review, protocol revisions, or adverse event reports) should have a specialized review form that leads the reviewer through the important information that must be evaluated and the important determinations that must be made. The purpose of this chapter is to give IRB members some basic guidelines for how they should communicate their review to the rest of the committee.

- Limit the initial summary of your review to one to two minutes.

It is difficult to follow a presentation that lasts more than one to two minutes. When an IRB member understands what should be evaluated in a review and prepares the review prior to the IRB meeting, it is rare that a comprehensive summary of the important issues should take more than two minutes. Remember that the purpose of an initial presentation is to summarize the important points of the IRB review. As explained below, the primary reviewers should complete their presentations before the discussion is opened to other committee members.

- Your presentation should consist of reading your review form.

As emphasized throughout this handbook, you should use a standardized review form to record all of the important information and determinations that are needed for IRB review of research protocols, revisions, and adverse event reports. If you use a good review form, and organize the information in writing before the meeting, your presentation to the committee will simply consist of reading your completed review form.

- Resist the urge to impress the committee with how much work you did.

It many situations, a high quality review requires many hours of hard work on the part of a primary reviewer. The review may include discussions with the principal investigator and consultants, the reading of related literature, and clarification of initially confusing protocol information. There is a natural tendency for the primary reviewer to want to impress colleagues by making them relive the trials and tribulations of the review experience.

It is important for IRB members to recognize that the committee expects and appreciates a thorough review on the part of each primary reviewer but that optimal IRB function requires only a bottom-line summary at the IRB meeting. This is not to say that IRB members should not explain the efforts that they went through to evaluate a protocol item or the complex issues that they encountered. It is both important and appropriate for primary reviewers to explain to the IRB committee and document on a review form the important relevant events, including significant time factors. However, it is possible to summarize this information in a way that gives the committee the facts needed to make an informed determination without making them relive the details of the reviewer's experience.

• Presentations by secondary reviewers should focus on areas of disagreement with previous reviewers.

When there is more than one primary reviewer assigned to an agenda item, all successive reviewers should focus the presentation of their review on the areas where they disagree with the previous reviewer(s). Subsequent reviewers should communicate their evaluations by going down the list of important issues to consider and stating whether they agree or disagree with the information that was presented by previous reviewers. If there is disagreement or there are different interpretations, this should be explained in detail to the committee.

• Do not allow questions until after all of the primary reviewers have made their presentations.

In many situations, IRB members will want to ask questions to clarify their understanding of a primary reviewer's summary presentation. The IRB will function optimally if the IRB meeting is structured so that all of the primary reviewers complete their summary presentations before comments or questions are allowed from other IRB members.

• End your presentation with a vote recommendation.

There are many situations where a primary reviewer wants to consider the opinions of other IRB members before finalizing a decision on how to vote on an agenda item. This is how the IRB should function, and all IRB members should keep an open mind throughout full-committee discussions. However, it will improve the IRB review process if all primary reviewers approach their assignments with a goal of being able to end their initial presentation with a recommendation for how the committee should vote on the item in question. All IRB members should understand that such recommendations should be viewed as preliminary assessments that are being included in the initial presentations to help committee members clarify their thinking on the important issues that are required to make a determination on the agenda item that is being discussed.

C H A P T E R 2-8

DECIDING HOW TO VOTE

ROBERT J. AMDUR AND LIZ BANKERT

Deciding How to Vote or Not to Vote

- Undertand the five vote options:

  1. Abstained from voting
  2. Approved as submitted
  3. Conditionally approved
  4. Not approved or disapproved
  5. Tabled

- Use these two guidelines to decide how to vote:

  1. Use the three ethical principles described in the Belmont Report to analyze and explain concerns about research procedures.
  2. Vote *No* unless you are convinced that you should vote *Yes*.

After the primary reviewers have presented their summaries and the full committee has discussed the agenda item, there comes a time when IRB members must each decide how they are going to vote. In some IRBs the chair determines when the discussion is sufficient to call for a vote while in others a vote call requires the support of at least two IRB members. The purpose of this chapter is to clarify the basic vote options (including abstaining from voting) and then to present some basic guidelines for ethical decision making in this setting.

VOTE OPTIONS, INCLUDING ABSTAINING FROM VOTING

When voting on an agenda item, IRB members have five options to choose from when recording their determination:

1. **Abstain from voting:** This means that the IRB member does not vote on the agenda item. There are only two reasons that an IRB member should abstain from voting: conflict of interest and insufficient information to make an informed determination.

   Conflict of interest: IRB members should recognize that in most settings there will be no specific policy that defines when they should or should not abstain from voting at an IRB meeting. Most IRBs require that members abstain from voting on a protocol for which they are listed as a principal or co-investigator. Some institutions have a policy that requires IRB members to abstain from voting on protocols in which they have a financial interest above a certain dollar amount in the research sponsor.

   In view of the lack of specific guidelines on abstaining from voting at an IRB meeting, members will frequently have to decide to abstain from voting because of concern about conflict of interest. A practical guideline is that IRB members who think that they have a conflict of interest that may bias their judgment in evaluating the item under consideration should abstain from voting.

   Insufficient information to make an informed determination: IRB members who do not have the basic information they need to make an informed determination should abstain from voting on the item in question. Having said this, it is important to understand that IRB members should not use the "insufficient information" factor to avoid making a contentious or controversial determination. There are many situations where IRB members must make difficult decisions in the face of uncertainty. The lack of definitive guidelines for how to vote on an IRB issue is no excuse for avoiding the responsibility of rendering a judgment in the form on an IRB determination. As a general guideline, the only time it is appropriate to abstain from voting based on insufficient information is when the IRB member was not present for the critical aspects of the discussion of an IRB issue.

2. **Approved as submitted:** This means that the investigator is not required to make any changes in the protocol or consent document. The IRB may suggest changes, but as long as the changes are not required then the "approve as submitted" determination is applicable.

3. **Conditionally approved:** This means that the protocol will be approved if specific changes are made or information is clarified as directed by the IRB. The situations where an IRB is permitted to use this option is currently controversial within the regulatory community. Many IRBs use this vote option only when the required changes can be explained in such detail that the investigator is told exactly what the change must be on a word-for-word basis.

4. **Not approved or disapproved:** This means that the IRB is not able to specify the conditions under which it would approve the protocol item at the time of the current meeting.

5. **Table:** Many IRBs include "table" as a voting option, even though it is not mentioned in federal research regulations or guidance documents. In the setting of an IRB meeting, a vote to table a protocol means that the committee requests additional information from the investigator. From the functional standpoint, a table determination means that the investigator is prohibited from starting the study. Common

reasons to table a protocol include the need to review the answers to questions raised by IRB members or the need to review the investigator's response to requested modifications.

SEMANTICS: TABLE, DISAPPROVE, AND NOT APPROVE

Since the procedural implications, in terms of starting or not starting the study, are the same for both the IRB and the investigator, some IRBs prefer to simplify the decision process at the IRB meeting by deleting "table" as a determination option. IRBs that do not give the committee the option of tabling a protocol simply determine if the protocol is approved, approved pending specific modifications (conditional approval), or not approved (disapproval). When a protocol is not approved, the letter to the investigator summarizes the reasons that the committee did not approve the protocol at the current meeting. The point is that the IRB does not need a table option to convey determinations to investigators or to administer the voting process. So, why do IRBs table protocols instead of simply not approving them?

IRBs who prefer to table rather than not approve a protocol explain that they are concerned about the psychological impact a "not approved" or "disapproved" determination may have on the investigator. The thinking is that "table" more clearly indicates that the protocol is still under evaluation by the IRB, whereas "not approve" or "disapprove" implies that the IRB objects to a fundamental aspect of the study. There is no limit to the extent one could debate this question of psychological impact. In our experience, investigators do not care about the label of the IRB determination. Investigators want to know if the protocol is or is not approved by the IRB, because this determines if they can start the study. When they are not permitted to start the study after the IRB meeting, the investigator wants to know why the study was not approved and what should be done to have the protocol reconsidered as soon as possible.

In some cases, an IRB might want to delete "table" from the determination options. In our experience removing this category from the list of potential IRB determinations simplifies the voting process and helps to clarify the functional implications of an IRB decision. The phrase "not approve" or "disapprove" tends to focus the committee on the next step in the dialogue with the investigator. When the IRB is unable to approve a study, it is essential that the committee articulate the reasons for this determination in a way that clearly indicates the information that the IRB needs to reconsider the study or the items to address if the investigator wishes to appeal the determination.

USING ETHICAL PRINCIPLES TO DETERMINE HOW TO VOTE

There will be many situations where it is difficult for IRB members to make decisions about how they should vote on a given IRB agenda item. The most common scenario is that an IRB member is concerned about some aspect of the protocol but is not sure if voting to "not approve" the item is justified.

The bottom line is that there is no way to eliminate the tension and uncertainty that is often associated with making IRB determinations. The nature of such work is that IRB members will frequently be required to make difficult decisions without definitive guidance that have major implications for investigators and/or subjects. Two guidelines will help IRB members structure their thinking on how to vote at the IRB meeting:

1. **Use the three ethical principles described in the Belmont Report to analyze and explain concerns about research procedures:** The Belmont Report, discussed in Chapter 1-4, presents the principles of respect for persons, beneficence, and justice—the tools that IRB members should use to analyze research procedures. It is much easier to evaluate the

important IRB issues and to explain concerns to
other IRB members if one has a language for discussing the ethical standards of research involving
human subjects. The Belmont Report gives IRB
members the language they need to explain why they
are concerned about a research procedure in a way
that gets to the core ethical issues and is consistent
from one discussion to another.

2. **Vote "No" unless you are convinced that you should
   vote "Yes":** This is another way of saying that IRB
   members should vote to not approve a protocol
   unless they are confident that they should vote to
   approve or conditionally approve the protocol.

The mission of the IRB is to protect the rights and
welfare of research subjects. IRB members should take
the approach that the information reviewed by the
IRB—including discussion at the IRB meeting—should
provide all the information that they need to feel that it
is acceptable to approve the protocol under discussion.
IRB members should never be told, or be permitted to
feel, that their concern about an issue should be ignored
because they don't understand the details of the situation.
IRB members do not need to understand complex scientific information or procedures to evaluate core ethical
issues. IRB members with expertise in the research under
discussion should be able to explain the research in a way
that all IRB members understand the important information. If IRB members do not understand the information they need to make an informed decision, they
should vote to not approve the protocol until they get
this level of understanding. Similarly, IRB members
should vote to not approve the protocol unless they feel
comfortable that the proposal protects the rights and
welfare of the subjects as much as possible.

PART 3

Specific
Topics

EVALUATING STUDY DESIGN AND QUALITY

ROBERT J. AMDUR

How the IRB Evaluates Study Design and Scientific Quality

Ethical codes and federal regulations require that the IRB evaluate the study design and scientific quality. For example:

- Section 18 of the Declaration of Helsinki (2000):

  Medical research involving human subjects should only be conducted if the importance of the objective outweighs the inherent risks and burdens to the subject.

- Federal Regulation 45 CFR 46.111(a):

  Criteria for IRB approval of Research: Risks to subjects are minimized by using procedures which are consistent with sound research design, and which do not, unnecessarily, expose subjects to risk.

It is not unusual for IRB members, institutional officials, and researchers to debate the role of the IRB in evaluating study design or other aspects that affect the fundamental quality of the science of research. For example, is it appropriate for IRB members to vote not to approve a study because they believe study results would be more persuasive if a different control group was used, or because previously completed research has already answered the study question? Is it appropriate for the

IRB to question the validity of the statistical power calculation used to determine the number of subjects in a study? Some members of the research community and some IRB members are under the impression that it is not the role of the IRB to routinely evaluate the "quality of the science" of a protocol. Many IRB chairs have been confronted with statements like "The IRB's job is to evaluate ethics. The IRB has no business commenting on the science of a study." In most cases this view will be presented by a researcher who has been criticized by the IRB, but in some situations the argument will come from IRB members or institutional officials.

The purpose of this chapter is to explain the role of the IRB in evaluating study design and the other features of a study that may affect scientific quality. The bottom line is that there is no question that the IRB not only has the authority to evaluate scientific quality, but it has the obligation to do so if it is to function in compliance with accepted ethical codes and federal research regulations.

ETHICAL CODES

Nuremberg Code (1949)

Several sections of the Nuremberg code address scientific quality and the risk/benefit profile. Point 3 is representative:

The experiment should be so designed and based on the results of animal experimentation and a knowledge of the natural history of the disease or other problem under study that the anticipated results will justify the performance of the experiment.

Declaration of Helsinki (2000)

Multiple sections of the latest version of this ethical code address specific aspects of study design. Sections 11, 18, and 29 are especially relevant to the question of IRB review of scientific quality:

11. Medical research involving human subjects must conform to generally accepted scientific principles and be based on a thorough knowledge of the scientific literature, other relevant sources of information, and adequate laboratory and, where appropriate, animal experimentation.

18. Medical research involving human subjects should only be conducted if the importance of the objective outweighs the inherent risks and burdens to the subject. This is especially important when the human subjects are healthy volunteers.

29. The benefits, risks, burdens, and effectiveness of a new method should be tested against those of the best current prophylactic, diagnostic, and therapeutic methods. This does not exclude the use of placebo, or no treatment, in studies where no proven prophylactic, diagnostic, or therapeutic method exists.

FEDERAL RESEARCH REGULATIONS

Department of Health and Human Services and corresponding Food and Drug Administration regulations require the IRB to determine that a study is designed so that risks to subjects are minimized and justified by potential benefits. For example, these guidelines are offered in 45 CFR 46.111(a) Criteria for IRB approval of Research:

(1) Risks to subjects are minimized: (i) by using procedures which are consistent with sound research design, and which do not, unnecessarily, expose subjects to risk.

THE IRB'S RESPONSIBILITY TO EVALUATE SCIENTIFIC QUALITY

The IRB is supposed to act in compliance with federal research regulations and make decisions that support the ethical principles in accepted ethical codes such as the Nuremberg Code and the Declaration of Helsinki. The sections from these guidance documents reproduced above emphasize that a characteristic of ethical research is that (1) the study is designed so that the risks to subjects are minimized and (2) the potential benefits of the research justify the potential risks. It is these two directives that establish the obligation of the IRB to carefully consider the study design and overall scientific quality of each study.

THE STUDY DESIGN

If revising the study design will meaningfully decrease the risk to subjects without a major compromise in the persuasiveness of the study results, then the IRB should not approve the protocol. Similarly, when a study that involves risk is set up to ask a question that is not important or has already been answered by previous research, the risk/benefit profile is likely to be unfavorable. The point is that the IRB is obligated to evaluate the study design and other aspects of scientific quality because these are ethical issues that affect the rights and welfare of research participants.

WHEN STUDY DESIGN IS SUBOPTIMAL BUT RISK IS MINIMAL

Having stressed the importance of evaluating the scientific quality of research, it is important to remember that as with all ethical principles, the IRB should use individual judgment and common sense when considering the rejection of a study based on problems with the study design. In organizations where a large volume of social science research is done by students, it is not unusual for the IRB to review protocols where the scientific design is not optimal but the risk to subjects is virtually zero.

Although one could argue that many of these student projects could legitimately be classified as educational exercises rather than research, that is a separate issue. The point is that there are projects where the study design is flawed, but the risk is basically zero. Certainly, it makes sense for IRB members who are knowledgeable in this type of research to recommend revisions to the study plan. However, in the absence of significant risk, there is really no ethical justification for the IRB to make such revisions a condition for IRB approval. Each case must be evaluated independently.

C H A P T E R 3-2

RESEARCHER CONFLICT OF INTEREST

DANIEL K. NELSON AND ROBERT J. AMDUR

Researcher Conflict of Interest

- For the purposes of IRB determinations, we can define a *conflict of interest* as a set of conditions in which an investigator's judgment concerning a primary interest (e.g., subject's welfare, integrity of research) may be biased by a secondary interest (e.g., personal gain).

- Saying that a conflict of interest exists does not mean that somebody made the wrong decision. It means that people who evaluate the situation may reasonably conclude that the potential for bias is such that improper decisions are possible.

- Disclosure to subjects does not, in and of itself, make a conflict of interest acceptable. Ethical research requires both disclosure *and* effective management of conflicts of interest.

- The IRB has several options for managing investigator conflict of interest:

  Prohibit conflicted investigators from having any involvement in the study.

  Prohibit conflicted investigators from participating in key components of the study—for example, the consent process, evaluation of inclusion criteria, specific procedures, and overall data analysis.

  Require a person who is not connected in any way to the investigator or study sponsor to act as a "subject advocate" during the initial and ongoing consent process.

Conflicts of interest (COI) are inherent to the conduct of research. In 1978 the National Commission for the Protection of Human Subjects of Biomedical and Behavioral Research wrote that "investigators are always in positions of potential conflict by virtue of their concern with the pursuit of knowledge as well as the welfare of the human subjects of their research." The commission echoed earlier reports by the National Institutes of Health (NIH) and the Surgeon General in viewing investigators as poorly positioned to reconcile these competing interests on their own, and in calling for a shared responsibility that incorporated independent review, such as the Institutional Review Board (IRB). The National Bioethics Advisory Commission (NBAC) reiterated this fundamental observation more than twenty years later in their current examination of the system of protections, noting that research "necessarily creates a conflict of interest for investigators" through their use of fellow humans to obtain knowledge. Note that neither commission held these conflicts to be irreconcilable, nor did they link conflict of interest to character flaws of investigators, as individuals or as a class. The goals of this chapter are to define conflict of interest and to discuss possible management strategies.

DEFINITIONS

Before considering conflicts of interest as they relate to research involving human subjects, it is important to establish a working definition. One source of confusion lies in the semantics of the discussion. The problem that we are trying to avoid is *bias in judgment.* We are looking for a term to describe situations where the potential for bias is such that decisions may be called into question. For the purposes of IRB determinations, a *conflict of interest* can be defined as a set of conditions in which an investigator's judgment concerning a primary interest (e.g., subject's welfare, integrity of research) may be biased by a secondary interest (e.g., personal gain).

One of the most misunderstood aspects of conflict of interest is that a problem exists even in the absence of documentation of bias or improper decisions. Saying that a conflict of interest exists does not mean that somebody made the wrong decision. It means that people who evaluate the situation may reasonably conclude that the potential for bias is such that improper decisions are likely. In other words, it is the people who evaluate the decision, not the person making the decisions, who determine if a conflict of interest exists. As P. J. Friedman explains, "a conflict exists whether or not decisions are affected by the personal interest; a conflict of interest implies only the potential for bias or wrongdoing, not a certainty or likelihood."

With regard to financial relationships, former *New England Journal of Medicine* editor Marcia Angell has defined conflict of interest as "any financial association that would cause an investigator to prefer one outcome … to another." Angell argues that there is no such thing as "potential" conflict of interest, since conflict is a function of the situation, not of the investigator's response to that situation. Thus the opportunity need not be acted on to represent a conflict of interest and a situation worthy of concern.

DISCLOSURE

In 1914 Supreme Court Justice Louis Brandeis wrote that "publicity is justly commended as a remedy for social and industrial diseases. Sunlight is said to be the best of disinfectants."

Disclosure to the Institution

Disclosure to the institution is mandatory for those investigators receiving federal funds, with their institutions given discretion in how they manage any conflicts. Predictably, there is considerable variability in how institutions handle this process. Many have established policies requiring disclosure by all faculty members.

However, few institutions have linked this process to protection of human subjects, as suggested by the fact that none of the 235 institutions in a recent survey incorporated disclosure to either IRBs or subjects as a management strategy in their conflict of interest policies.

Disclosure to the IRB

Disclosure to the IRB is increasingly advocated as a routine part of protocol review. OHRP has strongly recommended that financial relationships be described when investigators submit IRB applications, and that IRBs should take into consideration the funding arrangements between sponsor and investigator institution. A recent survey of 200 IRBs that oversee clinical trials suggests that only 25 percent review such financial matters. These have tended to be regarded, by both investigators and IRBs, as "none of our business." However, if IRBs are to fulfill their responsibility to protect research subjects from bias related to conflict of interest, they must evaluate the financial and other incentives that motivate the conduct of studies they review.

Disclosure to Subjects

Disclosure via the informed consent process is at once the most direct and ethically intuitive route of disclosure, but also the most difficult to accomplish in a meaningful way. At the very least, subjects should be aware that the study is sponsored by outside entities, be they commercial or governmental. As to the level of detail provided, we stop short of recommending that consent forms routinely include dollar amounts, even when investigators are paid on a per capita basis. Dollar amounts may be misleading, because some may represent justifiable expenses, some may represent inappropriate incentives, and some may be both at the same time.

A major misunderstanding for IRBs and investigators is the concept that full disclosure to subjects makes a conflict of interest acceptable. This is not the case. Ethical research requires both disclosure *and* effective management of conflicts of interest. IRBs must not "pass the buck" to subjects by shirking their responsibility to evaluate the possibility that conflicts will bias judgments in the conduct or analysis of research. It is well documented that research subjects often do not understand this kind of information beyond a superficial level. The principle of beneficence requires that the IRB not approve a study when there is a conflict of interest that is likely to bias judgment to a meaningful degree, regardless of the extent to which the conflict is explained in the consent process.

BEYOND DISCLOSURE

Management strategies should be aimed at eliminating or minimizing the conflict of interest. While IRBs may not be well situated or equipped to directly oversee this process, they should establish open lines of communication with those institutional bodies that are (for example, the Conflict of Interest Committee). IRBs should then consider the mechanisms proposed to manage the identified conflict, with a particular eye for aspects that could affect research subjects. The IRB has several options for managing investigator conflict of interest in the context of a given study:

- Prohibit conflicted investigators from having any involvement in the study.

- Prohibit conflicted investigators from participating in key components of the study—for example, the consent process, evaluation of inclusion criteria, specific procedures, and overall data analysis.

- Require a person who is not connected in any way to the investigator or study sponsor to act as a "subject advocate" during the initial and ongoing consent process.

Given that even the appearance of impropriety is enough to damage individual careers and institutional reputations, a cautious approach to these issues is in everyone's mutual interest. IRBs may first need to overcome the perception that managing conflict of interest is reliant on their trust of the investigator in question. Management should hinge not on anyone's perception of an individual but on an objective assessment of situations in which people have placed themselves. All parties involved in this process should be clear that managing conflict of interest has everything to do with the situation, and nothing to do with the character or honesty of the individual under question.

CHAPTER 3-3

ADVERTISEMENTS FOR RESEARCH

RACHEL HOMER, RACHEL KREBS, AND
LINDA MEDWAR

Advertisements for Research

The IRB must approve all plans for advertisement
(including the actual posters, brochures, scripts for
commercials, etc.) prior to their use. A 1998 update of
the FDA information sheet: *Recruiting Study Subjects*
presents guidelines for the format of study advertisement:

- Name and address of the investigator and/or
  research facility/institution
- Condition under study and/or purpose of the
  research
- Inclusion/exclusion criteria in summary form
- A brief list of procedures involved
- Time or other commitment required (number of
  visits, total duration including follow-up visits, etc.)
- Compensation/reimbursement
- Location of research and contact person for further
  information

Additional guidelines include the following:

- Advertisements should not emphasize monetary
  compensation.
- Advertisements should not use catchy words like
  "free" or "exciting."
- Advertisements should be very clear that *research*
  participation is what is being solicited.
- Advertisements should not be misleading about the
  purpose of the research.

The recruitment of subjects, which is considered the start of the consent/assent process, and the feasibility of recruiting must be considered and planned before initiation of a study and must continue throughout the study. For this reason, the IRB must review the methods, materials, procedures, and tools used to recruit potential research subjects before they are implemented. Some of the more commonly used tools of recruitment include direct advertising (flyers, posters, press releases, brochures), media advertisements (newspaper, TV, radio, websites), recruitment letters, review of medical charts and computerized databases, and presentations at community meeting places.

A 1998 update of the FDA information sheet *Recruiting Study Subjects* presents quidelines for the format of study advertisement:

- Name and address of the investigator and/or research facility/institution
- Condition under study and/or purpose of the research
- Inclusion/exclusion criteria in summary form
- A brief list of procedures involved
- Time or other commitment required (number of visits, total duration including follow-up visits, etc.)
- Compensation/reimbursement
- Location of research and contact person for further information

FLYERS, POSTERS, AND BROCHURES

Flyers, posters, and brochures are often used to solicit potential research subjects. These types of advertisements are typically placed in strategic locations in the hope of targeting the population being studied. Some of these locations may include bulletin boards, professional offices/businesses, schools, public transportation (buses, subways, trains), and public areas such as restaurants. While it is mandatory to obtain IRB approval for use of such advertisements, it may also be necessary for an investigator to obtain approval from the various sites where the flyer, poster, and/or brochure will be placed. This should also be done prior to posting or distribution of the ad, and evidence of this approval may be required by the IRB. Since these types of advertisements are visible tools of recruitment, they must present sufficient information that is accurate and balanced so that potential subjects are able to make an informed decision about possible participation. The decision to include compensation and/or reimbursement in the advertisement may be made on a case by case basis, depending on the study itself and the particular policies and guidelines of the IRB. Although compensation or reimbursement may factor into one's decision to participate in a study, it must be carefully thought out and worded appropriately so as not to coerce a subject to participate. The examples of acceptable and unacceptable research advertisements presented here will clarify these issues.

Example 1 presents an advertisement that should not be approved by the IRB. Several problems can be seen in this advertisement:

Lose Weight Fast and Receive Cash!!!

Join an Exciting Weight Loss Study

• *Are you a teenager?*

• *Are you fat and want to lose weight?*

If you answered YES to these questions, you may qualify to participate in a weight loss study.

You will receive a free medical evaluation and participate in a cutting-edge nutrition program. You will also receive $$$ money $$$ and parking vouchers. No medications will be given.

Call **(213) 456-9870** for more information.

Example 1: Unapproved Advertisement

- Monetary compensation is emphasized.
- Catchy words such as "exciting," "fast," "cutting-edge," and "free" are used.
- The ages for eligibility are not specified.
- The purpose of the study is not specified.
- There is no mention that this study is "research."
- Terms such as "fat" may be insulting.
- The name of contact person is not included.
- The study location is not included.
- The purpose of the advertisement is misleading.

This is an example of an advertisement that meets the basic guidelines for IRB approval:

***

Weight Loss and Diabetes Prevention Study

Be part of an important nutrition research study

- *Are you between 13 and 21 years of age?*
- *Do you want to change your eating habits in order to lose weight?*

If you answered YES to these questions, you may be eligible to participate in a nutrition research study.

The purpose of this research study is to compare the effectiveness of different diets in preventing Type 2 diabetes. Benefits include a comprehensive medical evaluation and nutrition program. Participation will also receive monetary compensation and parking vouchers. No medications will be given.

Both adolescents (13 years of age and older) and adults (21 years of age and younger) are eligible.

The study is being conducted at Central Hospital.

Please call Beth Woods at **(213) 456-9870** for more information.

***

Example 2: Revised Advertisement

- The approach is straightforward and honest.
- The type of research is specified.
- The ages for eligibility are included.
- The purpose is clearly stated.
- The benefits are included.
- The contact person's name is included.
- The institution is identified.

CHAPTER 3-4

DENYING SUBJECTS ACCESS TO RESEARCH RESULTS

THOMAS KEENS AND ROBERT J. AMDUR

Denying Subjects Access to Research Results

- Ethical research requires that, at the time of the initial consent process, subjects understand the conditions under which they will, or will not, be given research results.

- When potentially devastating results may be given to the subject, professional counseling should be part of the initial consent process to be sure that subjects understand the implications of their decision to participate in the study and/or to receive research results.

- The predictive value of research results is a critical factor in evaluating the ethics of the plan for subject access to research results.

- When informing subjects of research results may cause serious social harm, the principle of beneficence may justify withholding information from subjects concerning research results.

When research involves testing of subjects for potential markers of disease, the IRB must evaluate the plans of the study for informing the subjects of research results. Some studies plan to give subjects research results whether they ask for them or not while others give subjects results only in specific situations.

ETHICAL PRINCIPLES

The Belmont principles of respect for persons and beneficence address the issue of informing subjects about
research results. At first glance, these principles appear to
present competing obligations.

Respect for Persons

The principle of respect for persons acknowledges the
freedom and dignity of every person. A person should be
able to choose what will and will not happen to him or
her. Respect for persons means that ethical research
requires subjects to understand the full implications of
their decision to participate in a study. There are two
ways one could apply the principle of respect for persons
to the question of informing subjects of research results.
One view might argue that respect for persons requires
that researchers give each subject the option of being
informed of research results, with a full explanation of
the potential implications of this decision. With this perspective, researchers would be ethically obligated to
report research results to any subject who wants them.

The alternative view interprets the principle of respect
for persons to mean that informed consent requires the
potential subjects to understand if they will or will not be
informed of research results. However, there is no ethical
justification for requiring result disclosure per se.
Subjects are not required to participate in research. It is
perfectly ethical to allow people to exercise their right as
autonomous agents to decline to participate in a research
study because they do not agree with the plan to limit
access to research results.

Beneficence

Beneficence can be defined as the obligation to maximize
potential benefits and minimize potential risks. One
should not injure a person, despite possible benefits to
others or to society. This principle argues that the inves-

tigators should provide a subject with research information if that information will maximize benefits or minimize risks to the subject.

However, beneficence also argues that the investigator should not inform the subject about research results if that information will cause harm. In some situations making the subject aware of research results is likely to cause the subject psychological distress, stigmatization, discrimination, or other forms of social harm. This is especially problematic when the predictive value of the result is uncertain. Therefore, as a generalization, for speculative information—meaning information that has not been proved to have clinical relevance to the subject—the principle of beneficence suggests that the investigator is not obligated to inform the research subject. Further, since providing subjects with this information may cause harm, one can make an argument that the investigator has an ethical obligation to withhold such information from the research subject.

RECOMMENDATIONS

As part of their review of human research protocols, IRBs must decide whether or not research information should be given to subjects. To help in this determination, the IRB should consider the following issues:

1. A complete understanding of the extent to which research results will be disclosed to the subjects and/or their physicians is an absolute requirement of ethical research.

2. When considering the ethics of withholding research results from study subjects, an important consideration is the level of certainty that this information will impact the diagnosis, management, or prognosis of the subject.

3. Disclosing research results to subjects may harm research subjects. Risks may be the dominant factor when the accuracy of research results are in question.

4. In some situations, it is appropriate for the research plan to allow the subjects to choose whether research results will be given to them or to their physician.

5. When potentially devastating research results may be given to the subject, professional counseling should be part of the initial consent process to be sure that subjects understand the implications of their decision to participate in the study and/or to receive research results.

PAYING RESEARCH SUBJECTS

BRUCE G. GORDON, JOSEPH BROWN,
CHRISTOPHER KRATOCHVIL,
ERNEST D. PRENTICE, AND ROBERT J. AMDUR

Paying Research Subjects

- The first thing to determine is if a payment is an *inducement* or a *reimbursement* (for direct expenses). There is no debate about the ethics of reimbursing subjects for direct expenses. Inducement payments are what the IRB is worried about.

- There are four basic models for paying research subjects:

  1. Market model: The laws of supply and demand determine how much a subject should be paid for participating in a given trial.
  2. Wage payment model: Payment is made based on the premise that participation in research is unskilled labor that requires little training and some risk. Thus subjects are compensated "on a scale commensurate with that of other unskilled but essential jobs"; that is, a fairly low, standardized hourly wage, with bonuses for hazardous procedures.
  3. Fair share model: Investigators are typically reimbursed a certain amount of money per patient. Utilizing this model, subjects would be compensated a fixed proportion of the per-subject reimbursement that is given to the investigator.
  4. Reimbursement model: The above three models accept the premise that it is ethically acceptable to use money to induce people to participate in research. In the reimbursement model, payment is only permitted to cover the subject's expenses (travel, food, gasoline, lost wages).

Payment of human subjects to participate in research remains one of the most contentious ethical problems facing IRBs. Though concerns over this practice have existed for many years, there are few regulatory guidelines, nor indeed any consensus to shape institutional and individual IRB policy. In this chapter, we will briefly review the ethical arguments pertaining to this practice, the federal regulations and guidance, and some of the models proposed to standardize the practice.

REIMBURSEMENT VERSUS INDUCEMENT

In order to evaluate the ethics of paying subjects for their participation in research, the first thing the IRB should do is determine if the payment is a reimbursement or an inducement. A payment is a *reimbursement* when it is meant to directly offset the direct, out-of-pocket costs that a subject incurs as a result of participating in the study. For example, in some studies subjects will end up paying for things like gas, parking, child care, or food to make the appointments that are required for the research procedures. In this case paying subjects an amount that basically offsets these direct expenses should be classified as a reimbursement for participating in research, not an inducement to participate in research.

In contrast, an *inducement* is a payment that is meant to motivate the subject to participate in the study for financial gain. A financial inducement to participate in research is a payment that is clearly greater than the expenses that a subject would be expected to incur to participate in the study. Some study applications explain that payment is being offered to compensate subjects for the time they will have to miss from work in order to participate in the study. If there are lost wages as a result of research participation, then a payment may be a reimbursement. However, if the subject is unemployed, or taking vacation time or sick time with pay, then there are no lost wages to reimburse.

The distinction between reimbursement and inducement payments is critical to the IRB evaluation process.

There is no ethical controversy about reimbursements for costs related to research participation regardless of the dollar amount of the payment, the risks of research participation, or the subject population. By definition, reimbursements do not coerce people into participating in research. Inducement payments are what the IRB is worried about, and it is this category of payment that the IRB must struggle with as it tries to determine where appropriate compensation ends and coercion begins.

PAYMENT FOR "INCONVENIENCE" IS AN INDUCEMENT, NOT A REIMBURSEMENT

Many published policies regarding the payment of research subjects, including some federal guidance documents, explain that it is acceptable to pay subjects for inconvenience and time spent in research participation as long as the payments are not so large as to induce prospective subjects to consent to participate in the research against their better judgment. In reading these kinds of directives, IRB members should understand that they often serve to confuse the distinction between inducement and reimbursement payments for research participation. Payment for inconvenience is an inducement to participate in research, not a reimbursement for incurred expenses. For this reason the arguments against inducement payments that are the subject of the next section apply to the use of financial incentives to get people to accept the inconvenience of participating in research.

ARGUMENTS AGAINST INDUCEMENT PAYMENTS FOR RESEARCH PARTICIPATION

Coercion

The main argument against using money or financial gain to induce people to participate in research is that such payments are coercive. The IRB should not approve research in which subjects are likely to be coerced into research participation because this "undue influence" violates the Belmont principle of respect for persons. This fundamental ethical standard requires that research participation be completely voluntary, which means free of coercion or undue influence.

Coercion is one of the most difficult issues for the IRB to evaluate because it is not possible to establish objective guidelines that define when a situation is, or is not, coercive. It has been said that coercion is kind of like pornography: difficult to define but you know it when you see it.

The rebuttal to the coercion argument is that it is unethically paternalistic for the IRB to prevent subjects from doing something that they want to do as long as they understand the implications of their decision. Inherent to this argument is the concept that payments to subjects represent a true benefit of research participation. While this may seem obvious to some people, it has been a confusing issue in the regulatory community because there is a guidance document from the Food and Drug Administration that specifically tells the IRB *not* to view subject payments as a benefit of research participation. This directive likely reflects a misunderstanding about the difference between reimbursement and inducement payments.

Inducement Payments Dehumanize Both Subject and Researcher

Another argument against paying research subjects is that such payment dehumanizes subjects and, by making them a "salaried worker," potentially alters the relationship between the subject and the investigator. Payment for participation in research amounts to selling the services of one's body, often at some significant risk.

This issue is complex because payment for labor is not fundamentally unethical; one's services or capacities are commodities that in our free-market social and economic system are regularly exchanged for wages. Nor would it generally be considered unethical to pay wages for work that is inherently risky (police, firefighters, and commercial fisherman regularly experience risk in their jobs). One might note that many would be uncomfortable with the notion of being paid for the risk per se. Some people argue that inducement payments for research participation are ethical because the payments are used to induce people to perform the job of a research subject and that the risk associated with that job is a secondary issue. Clearly the distinction between the job of being a research subject and the risk associated with that job is a nebulous concept that is difficult for the IRB to use in making determinations.

One could write an entire book on the issue of paying for research participation. The final point to make here is that many of the issues involved in evaluating the ethics of research payments mirror those of the debate about legalizing prostitution. Some ethicists argue that using money to induce people to participate in research is no different than paying for prostitution because what is being bought and sold in prostitution, just as in participation in research, is something that is "so intimate to one's person that there is something disturbing in the notion that it is alienable, as a commodity." The ethical objections to prostitution, and to being a paid-research subject, derive from the translation of relations that are supposed to express fundamental aspects of humanity into an economic exchange. In the paid research context, both the investigator and the subject are reducing an essential human capacity (putting oneself at risk for others) to a commodity. In so doing, they may dehumanize each other.

Inducement Payments Violate the Belmont Principle of Justice

The final argument related to inducement payments for research is the concern that such payment is likely to result in economically disadvantaged persons bearing a disproportionately large share of the risks of research and thereby to violate the Belmont principle of justice.

However, it has been asserted that this view is rather one-sided because it considers research solely as a "burden." To the extent that the benefits of research are distributed primarily to participants, one might argue that any procedure such as payment of subjects that encourages recruitment of populations that have traditionally not participated in clinical research, like African Americans, is ethically acceptable and appropriate. Of course, this argument is based on the assumption that participation in the research is undoubtedly beneficial. Members of minority populations would clearly disagree with that assumption or they would participate without inducement. Certainly, historical abuses such as the Tuskegee Study suggest that a certain suspicion of the research community is not without foundation.

MODELS FOR PAYMENT

IRBs that ultimately decide to allow payment to research subjects must decide what level of compensation is appropriate. The literature on this subject describes four basic models for paying research subjects: (1) market model, (2) wage payment model, (3) fair share model, and (4) reimbursement model.

Market Model

In this model, the laws of supply and demand determine how much a subject should be paid for participating in a given trial. Payment is a "benefit" to offset risks associated with a particular trial. Studies that involve greater risk (or have no other benefit) would likely have the highest rate of compensation. Studies in which subjects stand to gain a significant health benefit (i.e., therapeutic studies) would likely have minimal or no monetary payment. This model also allows for higher compensation to speed recruitment, and bonuses to ensure that subjects complete the study.

Wage Payment Model

In this model, payment is made based on the premise that participation in research is unskilled labor that requires little training and some risk. Thus subjects are compensated "on a scale commensurate with that of other unskilled but essential jobs"—that is, a fairly low, standardized hourly wage, with bonuses for hazardous procedures.

Fair Share Model

In this model, the subject is treated like a partner in the research enterprise rather than a commodity or a wage laborer. Investigators are typically reimbursed a certain amount of money per patient. This is then used by the investigator to pay the direct (e.g., lab fees, IV tubing) and indirect (e.g., salaries, overhead) costs associated with performance of the study at his location. Utilizing this model, subjects would be compensated a fixed proportion of the per-subject reimbursement. Since investigator reimbursement per patient is based in part on whether a subject completes the trial, subjects' compensation would thus be prorated depending on the duration of their participation.

Reimbursement Model

The above three models accept the premise that it is ethically acceptable to use money to induce people to participate in research. The market, wage, and fair share models differ only in how they value the concern about paternalism, coercion, dehumanization, and justice as discussed in the preceding section. The reimbursement model of subject payment takes the stand that there is no situation in which it is ethical to use inducement payments to motivate people to participate in research.

In the reimbursement model, payment is provided to cover a subject's expenses (travel, food, gasoline). The definition of "expenses" may be somewhat flexible and can, at one end of the spectrum, be considered to include lost wages resulting from time taken off from work without pay. This model is based on the view that "research participation should not require financial sacrifice but should be revenue neutral for participants."

PRORATING PAYMENT

The FDA clearly requires a system of prorating payments based on the duration of participation of the subject in the research. The FDA information sheets state, "Any credit for payment should accrue as the study progresses and not be contingent upon the subject completing the entire study." Prorated payment should be made regardless of whether withdrawal was voluntary or involuntary—that is, whether the withdrawal was based on the decision of the subject to discontinue or based on some withdrawal criterion of the research protocol.

C H A P T E R 3 · 6

DECEPTION OF RESEARCH SUBJECTS

LAURIE SLONE, JAY HULL, AND
ROBERT J. AMDUR

Deception of Research Subjects

The American Psychological Association (APA) has developed guidelines for the conduct of research that involves deception of subjects:

- Psychologists never deceive research participants about significant aspects that would affect their willingness to participate, such as physical risks, discomfort, or unpleasant emotional experiences.

- Any other deception that is an integral feature of the design and conduct of an experiment must be explained to participants as early as is feasible—preferably, at the conclusion of their participation, but no later than at the conclusion of the research.

Providing Participants with Information About the Study

- If scientific or humane values justify delaying or withholding this information, psychologists take reasonable measures to reduce the risk of harm.

The following guidelines should be applied to the consent document:

- The consent document should never be used as part of the deception and thus should not include anything that is untrue.

- The consent document should reveal as much as possible to the participant regarding the procedures in the study.

- The consent document need not explain the details of the study if this will eliminate the capability of the study to inform the process under investigation.

The purpose of this chapter is to discuss research in which the subject is intentionally deceived about research participation. Deception is common in studies that evaluate fundamental aspects of human behavior. The rationale for deception in this setting is that it is not possible to obtain accurate information about how people behave when they know that they are being observed or evaluated.

GUIDELINES FOR RESEARCH INVOLVING DECEPTION

If one grants that it is impossible to study certain aspects of human behavior without adopting deceptive techniques, then the justification of such research evolves into a question of costs and benefits: the benefits gained by knowledge relative to the potential harm caused by deception. To some extent, this is a question of personal values. However, it also suggests that specific codes of conduct should be developed that serve to minimize the negative impact of deceptive techniques. The American Psychological Association (APA) has developed such a code. The two sections relevant to deception in research read as follows:

6.15   Deception in Research

a. Psychologists do not conduct studies involving deception unless they have determined that the use of deceptive techniques is justified by the study's prospective scientific, educational, or applied value. In addition, they have determined that equally effective alternative procedures that do not use deception are not feasible.

b. Psychologists never deceive research participants about significant aspects that would affect their willingness to participate, such as physical risks, discomfort, or unpleasant emotional experiences.

c. Any other deception that is an integral feature of the design and conduct of an experiment must be explained to participants as early as is feasible—preferably, at the conclusion of their participation, but no later than at the conclusion of the research.

6.18 Providing Participants with Information About the Study

a. Psychologists provide a prompt opportunity for participants to obtain appropriate information about the nature, results, and conclusions of the research, and psychologists attempt to correct any misconceptions that participants may have.

b. If scientific or humane values justify delaying or withholding this information, psychologists take reasonable measures to reduce the risk of harm.

According to the APA, deception in research basically requires that the researcher (1) apply a cost/benefit analysis that explicitly considers the potential for harm created and/or exacerbated by the use of deception; (2) consider alternative methodologies; and (3) fully explain the nature of the deception at the conclusion of the study or explicitly justify withholding such information. In all cases, the safety and comfort of the participant should be of paramount concern.

GUIDELINES FOR THE CONSENT DOCUMENT

By definition, deceptive procedures eliminate the possibility of fully informed consent. As a consequence, the APA code makes this explicit statement: "Psychologists never deceive research participants about significant aspects that would affect their willingness to participate." Although participants may not be fully informed, obviously they should be informed of as much as possible without threatening the ability of the researcher to test the true hypothesis of the study. Our recommendation is that the IRB should not approve a consent document that contains inaccurate information. Specifically:

- The consent document should *never* be used as part of the deception and thus should not include anything that is untrue.

- The consent document should reveal as much as possible to the participant regarding the procedures in the study.

- The consent document need not explain the details of the study if this will eliminate the capability of the study to inform the process under investigation. A useful guideline to keep in mind is that the experimenter–subject relationship is a real relationship "in which we have responsibility toward the subject as another human being whose dignity we must preserve."

QUALITATIVE SOCIAL SCIENCE RESEARCH

DEAN R. GALLANT AND ROBERT J. AMDUR

Qualitative Social Science Research

- Informed consent is an important part of qualitative research. Much qualitative research is exploratory, and the areas of inquiry may not be apparent even to the research team at the time the study is initiated. Qualitative research should be designed to sustain the consent process throughout the course of a subject's participation.

- Qualitative researchers may encounter reportable situations—evidence of child or elder abuse or neglect, or the likely prospect of harm to self or others. In most states, investigators have a legal obligation to report such situations to appropriate authorities. Researchers who are at all likely to uncover reportable situations must be prepared for the possibility. Appropriate consultation should be available if the researcher is not a trained clinician with relevant clinical experience. The IRB should consider the adequacy of the investigator's plans and may want to seek counsel from experts in the field.

- If identifiers must be retained (for longitudinal studies, or where subjects are videotaped or audiotaped), and if the research deals with very sensitive topics, it may be appropriate to seek a certificate of confidentiality to protect against compelled disclosure—by federal, state, or local authorities—of identifying information.

Not all research in the social sciences is laboratory-based experimental work. There is a long tradition of *qualitative research* by anthropologists, ethnographers, sociologists, survey researchers, psychologists, and others whose observations are typically conducted outside the laboratory. The purpose of their research is often to *develop* hypotheses rather than to test and validate them in controlled studies. Methods include observation (including participant observation), questionnaires or surveys, interviewing, or review and analysis of existing data. Because of the potential range of activities involved, qualitative research in the social sciences can present special problems for IRBs, for investigators, and for the subjects themselves.

TYPES OF RISK IN QUALITATIVE RESEARCH

Breach of Confidentiality

Subjects routinely share the stories of their daily lives with friends and colleagues. But, typically, a researcher collects information with the hope of publishing the results—if not necessarily attributing the subjects' comments directly (as a reporter might do), then at least revealing the cumulative knowledge gained from the research inquiry. If identities are poorly disguised, whether from others or from the participants themselves, subjects can risk embarrassment or more serious harm.

Violation of Privacy

Privacy refers to a state of being free from unsanctioned intrusion. Ordinarily, individuals have a right to privacy—that is, control over the extent, timing, and circumstances of sharing information about themselves with others. Violation of this right, although not necessarily a direct harm, contradicts the Belmont Report's principle of respect for persons.

Validation of Bad Behavior

Some research may unintentionally reinforce undesirable characteristics of research subjects. An investigator interviewing members of clandestine militant groups in a war-torn country worried about his ability to collect good data, thinking that subjects would be unwilling to reveal their "secrets." But to his surprise, and perhaps dismay, subjects reported that this interest from a faculty member at a major research institution gave an imprimatur of legitimacy to their anarchistic efforts! Another investigator studying recreational drug use among teens quickly learned it was necessary to develop a relationship of trust with his subjects, including being able to talk with them without criticizing their drug-taking behavior. A non-judgmental relationship like this, with a senior researcher at a prominent university, can have the unhappy effect of persuading subjects that their behavior is acceptable—if not fascinating—to wise adults. In such cases, it may be appropriate for the IRB to discuss its concerns with the investigator to help narrow the gap between strict scientific objectivity and responsible social values.

Risk of Harm to Others

Are possible harms to *secondary research subjects*—that is, individuals who do not themselves participate in the study but about whom the investigator obtains information via interview or other hearsay means—an appropriate area of concern for the IRB? In December 1999, the Office of Protection from Research Risks cited failure to obtain informed consent from secondary subjects as a finding in a letter of suspension of IRB authority. Oral historians and genetics researchers, among others, reacted promptly, insisting that extension of this regulatory interpretation would effectively halt much of their research, since they could not possibly obtain informed consent from everybody about whom they indirectly received information. As of this writing, the question is unresolved, but OPRR (now Office of Human Research

Protection [OHRP]) has not rescinded its interpretation, so IRBs should at least consider whether special consideration should be given to secondary subjects in studies where primary informants provide information about others.

INFORMED CONSENT

Although the content and issues may differ, informed consent is no less important in qualitative research than it is in clinical research. However, much qualitative research is exploratory, and the areas of inquiry may not be apparent even to the research team. How then can subjects truly be informed? Prior information about risks, insofar as they are known or can be anticipated, cannot be withheld. But if the range of possible risks is potentially very large, how can an investigator present accurate information about the study in a manner that will not simply frighten subjects away? One strategy is to sustain the consent process throughout the course of a subject's participation. As new data are acquired, and the researcher's overall knowledge of risks expands, subjects can be reminded that participation is voluntary, and their understanding of the risks and benefits of participation can be refreshed. This process should not be used to mask risks, nor to lure subjects into a relationship with the investigator before they fully understand the consequences, but it can help them develop an understanding of the research and the context of their role in it. Their continued participation is then based on active awareness of emerging developments.

REPORTABLE SITUATIONS

Much qualitative research deals with sensitive topics and looks deeply into subjects' daily lives. As a result, investigators may encounter reportable situations: evidence of child or elder abuse or neglect, or the likely prospect of harm to self or others. In most states, investigators have a legal obligation to report such situations to appropriate authorities. Researchers who are at all likely to uncover reportable situations must be prepared for the possibility. Appropriate consultation should be available if the researcher is not a trained clinician with relevant clinical experience. A strategy for alerting subjects to the need for reporting is essential; depending on the nature of the study and the subject population, this can involve mention of the reporting requirement as part of the informed consent process, or a more ad hoc procedure when the likelihood of reportable situations is small. The IRB should consider the adequacy of the investigator's plans and may want to seek counsel from experts in the field.

CERTIFICATE OF CONFIDENTIALITY

Whether or not a researcher is studying behaviors likely to yield information about reportable situations, subjects' reputations, relationships, employability, or legal status may be threatened by disclosure of identifiable information. The law does not recognize any automatic privilege for social science researchers; data are vulnerable to subpoena or other official inquiry. If identifiers must be retained (for longitudinal studies, or where subjects are videotaped or audiotaped), and if the research deals with very sensitive topics, it may be appropriate to seek a certificate of confidentiality to protect against compelled disclosure—by federal, state, or local authorities—of identifying information. Certificates of confidentiality can be granted by the federal funding agency, upon application, and are also available to investigators without federal funding. These certificates do not prohibit the investigator from disclosing information (and, in some states, confidentiality certificate protections are overridden by mandated reporting requirements), but they do provide a measure of protection for research subjects that would not otherwise be available.

CHAPTER 3-8

RESEARCH WITHOUT INFORMED CONSENT OR DOCUMENTATION

MARIANNE M. ELLIOT AND ROBERT J. AMDUR

Research Without Informed Consent or Documentation Thereof

Requirements to waive the requirement for informed consent:

- The research involves no more than minimal risk to the subjects.

- The waiver or alteration will not adversely affect the rights and welfare of the subjects.

- The research could not practicably be carried out without the waiver or alteration.

- Whenever appropriate, the subjects will be provided with additional pertinent information after participation.

Circumstances when an IRB may waive the requirement for <u>documentation</u> of informed consent:

- The only record linking the subject and the research would be the consent document, and the principal risk would be potential harm resulting from a breach of confidentiality. Each subject will be asked whether the subject wants documentation linking the subject with the research, and the subject's wishes will govern.

- The research presents no more than minimal risk of harm to subjects and involves no procedures for which written consent is normally required outside of the research context.

The purpose of this chapter is to explain the situations where federal regulations permit the IRB to approve research and waive the requirement for informed consent or the requirement for documentation of informed consent. A special case of the waiver of consent issue is the situation where research is conducted without consent in the setting of a medical emergency. There is an extensive list of requirements for IRB approval of research in the setting of a medical emergency that are described in federal regulations that were established specifically to deal with this controversial situation. The discussion in this chapter does not apply to the situation where research is conducted without consent in the setting of a medical emergency.

REQUIREMENTS FOR AN IRB TO WAIVE THE REQUIREMENT FOR INFORMED CONSENT (45 CFR 46.116 [D])

An IRB may approve a consent procedure that does not include, or which alters, some or all of the elements of informed consent set forth in this section, or waive the requirement to obtain informed consent provided the IRB finds and documents the following:

- The research involves no more than minimal risk to the subjects.

- The waiver or alteration will not adversely affect the rights and welfare of the subjects.

- The research could not practicably be carried out without the waiver or alteration.

- Whenever appropriate, the subjects will be provided with additional pertinent information after participation.

Example 1

The researcher plans to determine how mood and perception of one's body image may be related. Initially subjects complete a series of written questionnaires and scales about their body image. After the subjects are presented with visual images intended to evoke a negative mood, the subjects are asked to complete the same questionnaires and scales. The effect of evoking a negative mood is evaluated.

Although the actual purpose of the research is to determine how mood may be related to body image, subjects are informed that the research is actually two separate research projects: one related to moods and how they may change and the other related to body image. This deception is part of the research design, and the student subjects are not fully informed about the purpose of the research.

In this example, the IRB may find that an alteration of informed consent is appropriate and that the criteria stated above have been met based on the following:

1. **The research involves minimal risk:** The visual images are similar to those that the subjects might see in magazines about health and exercise, or movies. There are no provocative images. The questionnaires and scales are valid and reliable scales that are used in standard psychosocial testing.

2. **The rights and welfare of subjects are not adversely affected:** Subjects are informed about the actual procedures of the research, the lack of anticipated benefits, and the ability to discontinue participation at any time without penalty. Subjects are not informed that the research actually has one purpose and that the data will be evaluated for that intent.

3. **The research could not practicably be carried out without the alteration in the informed consent process:** The research evaluates a feature of human behavior that is likely to be affected by the subjects' knowledge of the behavior that is being evaluated.

4. **In this research, it is appropriate to provide subjects with additional pertinent information after participation.** The researcher debriefs the subjects after their participation to explain the actual purpose of the research and why the research design was appropriate. The researcher also offers to be available for any questions subjects may have and provides information about appropriate services if subjects experience distress or anxiety about their participation in the research.

Example 2

The researcher plans to determine whether some specific blood chemistry values change in individuals undergoing clinically indicated abdominal surgery and if there is a correlation of changes with the increased incidence of complications after surgery. The researcher plans to review the medical records of all individuals who have undergone abdominal surgery in the past year and for the next year. From a preliminary estimate, there are about 1,000 abdominal surgeries performed per year at the hospital. The researcher will collect limited data for this for research. The types of data to be collected include such items as the diagnosis before surgery, the type of abdominal surgery, specific blood chemistry values before the surgery, the same specific blood chemistry values after the surgery, a description of problems after surgery, and perhaps the age ranges of the individuals. The researcher will double-code the data so that the link is known only to the researcher and no others, in the unlikely event the data must be verified for accuracy. The results of the research will not affect the clinical care of the individuals, as the information will not be examined until after subjects leave the hospital.

In this example the IRB may find that a waiver of informed consent is appropriate and that the criteria stated above have been met based on the following:

1. **The research involves minimal risk:** The review of medical records is for limited information, the information is not sensitive in nature, and the data are

derived from clinically indicated procedures. The precautions taken to limit the record review to specified data and the double coding of the data further minimize the major risk, which is a breach of confidentiality.

2. **The rights and welfare of the individual would not be adversely affected:** The clinically indicated surgical procedure and the associated blood chemistry values were already completed, or would be completed, regardless of the research.

3. **The research could not be practicably carried out without the waiver:** Identifying and contacting the thousands of potential subjects, while not impossible, would not be feasible to get consent to review medical records.

4. **Providing subjects with additional information is not appropriate:** It would not be appropriate to provide these subjects with additional pertinent information about the results of the research as the results would have no effect on the subjects.

REQUIREMENTS FOR AN IRB TO WAIVE THE REQUIREMENT FOR DOCUMENTATION OF INFORMED CONSENT (45 CFR 46.117 [C])

Federal regulations describe two circumstances when an IRB may waive the requirement to obtain a signed consent form:

- The only record linking the subject and the research would be the consent document, and the principal risk would be potential harm resulting from a breach of confidentiality. Each subject will be asked whether the subject wants documentation linking the subject with the research, and the subject's wishes will govern.

- The research presents no more than minimal risk of harm to subjects and involves no procedures for which written consent is normally required outside of the research context.

In cases in which the documentation requirement is waived, the IRB may require the investigator to provide subjects with a written statement regarding the research.

Example 3

A researcher plans to evaluate the effectiveness of a smoking cessation program with women who are receiving prenatal care at the local health clinic. During a prenatal visit, any women who are already participating in the smoking cessation program will be asked to complete a written questionnaire about the program. The one-time written questionnaire includes questions about how well the women are complying with the program and how they feel about their progress. There is no identifying information about subjects on the questionnaire, and whether the subjects complete the questionnaire has no effect on the care they may receive at the clinic.

In this example, the IRB may waive the requirement to obtain a signed consent form because the research presents no more than minimal risk of harm to subjects. The questionnaire has no identifying information about the subject, and the purpose of the research is to evaluate the effectiveness of the program itself. Normally, there is no requirement for written consent for completion of written questionnaires outside the research context. By virtue of completing the questionnaire, subjects have consented to participate in the research. In this case, the IRB may require the researcher to provide subjects with a written summary or an information sheet about the research.

Example 4

A researcher plans face-to-face interviews with university students who belong to a support group on campus for trans- gendered, gay, lesbian, and bisexual individuals. The purpose of the research is to evaluate the quality of health care services for these individuals. The researcher plans to recruit subjects through flyers and information distributed at sup-

port group meetings. Potential subjects will contact the researcher directly. The researcher plans to conduct two face-to-face interviews six months apart. The interviews will be audiotaped, and the researcher will ask subjects to use a pseudonym during the interviews. Also, each subject will be assigned a coded number on the audiotape.

In this example, the IRB determines that the only record linking the subject and the research would be the consent document. The principal risk would be potential harm resulting from a breach of confidentiality if the consent documents were disclosed, purposefully or inadvertently. To minimize the potential harm to subjects, the IRB may permit the informed consent process to be conducted verbally and have the researcher document, perhaps in a research note, the circumstances of the consent process. The IRB may then request that the researcher ask subjects whether they want documentation linking them with the research, and each subject's wishes will be honored. The IRB may also require the researcher to provide each subject with a written summary or information sheet about the research. However, in this example, even having an information sheet about the research could be potentially harmful to subjects who may already suffer from social stigma, embarrassment, or ostracism. The IRB may suggest providing subjects with a card with only the name and phone number of the researcher in the event they have any questions or concerns.

It may be useful for the IRB to require that the investigator inform each subject about the temporal aspects of the risks associated with a signed consent document as the only link between the subject and the research. Subjects, as students or activists, might feel that the immediate potential harm from having a document with their signature confirming their participation in the research is minimal and a potential breach of confidentiality is not relevant. In contrast, the same subjects may find that the harm caused by an inadvertent breach of confidentiality perhaps five to ten years later during a job interview to be greater.

C H A P T E R 3 - 9

PASSIVE CONSENT (NOT SAYING NO)

LINDA J. KOBOKOVICH, ROBERT J. AMDUR,
AND ELIZABETH A. BANKERT

Research That Uses a Passive Consent Process

To approve the use of passive consent an IRB must
determine that the research meets either the regulatory
criteria for waiver of the requirement for informed consent or documentation thereof.

**Requirements for an IRB to waive the requirement
for informed consent:**

- The research involves no more than minimal risk to
  the subjects.
- The waiver or alteration will not adversely affect the
  rights and welfare of the subjects.
- The research could not practicably be carried out
  without the waiver or alteration.
- Whenever appropriate, the subjects will be provided
  with additional pertinent information after participation.

Circumstances when an IRB may waive the requirement for documentation of informed consent:

- The only record linking the subject and the research
  would be the consent document and the principal
  risk would be potential harm resulting from a
  breach of confidentiality. Each subject will be asked
  whether the subject wants documentation linking
  the subject with the research, and the subject's
  wishes will govern.
- The research presents no more than minimal risk of
  harm to subjects and involves no procedures for
  which written consent is normally required outside
  of the research context.

In organizations that conduct research involving survey interviews, the collection of information from the medical record, or the study of children at school, the IRB may encounter the situation where the investigator requests that the study be conducted based on the use of passive consent.   For the purposes of this discussion, *passive consent* is defined as a situation where the lack of an objection to research participation is considered to be an affirmative declaration of informed consent. This is a complicated way of saying that passive consent means that if you do not say "no," it means that you say "yes."

Example 1

A research study involves a survey that evaluates alcoholic beverage consumption in junior high school students. The survey will be administered in the school cafeteria during the student lunch break. The researchers will explain the essential elements of informed consent to potential subjects, and their assent is a requirement for study participation. The researchers have permission to conduct the study from the school principal. The researchers plan to inform parents of the study by sending them a letter at home that explains the study in detail. The letter explains that students will not be approached about the study if parents send in a "refusal to participate" card; the stamped, self-addressed card is included with the letter. The letter explains that if parents do not register an objection to the study, it will be assumed that they are giving the researchers permission to ask their child to participate.

In this example the researchers are asking the IRB to approve the study with the understanding that parental permission will be obtained using a passive procedure. To evaluate this issue, it is important that the IRB understand that to approve the use of a passive consent procedure, an IRB that operates in compliance with federal regulations must determine that the study meets either the criteria to waive the requirement for informed consent or the criteria to waive the requirement for documentation of informed consent.

The following requirements must be met for an IRB to waive the requirement for informed consent (45 CFR 46.116 [d]):

- The research involves no more than minimal risk to the subjects.

- The waiver or alteration will not adversely affect the rights and welfare of the subjects.

- The research could not practicably be carried out without the waiver or alteration.

- Whenever appropriate, the subjects will be provided with additional pertinent information after participation.

There are two circumstances when an IRB may waive the requirement for documentation of informed consent (45 CFR 46.117 [c]):

- The only record linking the subject and the research would be the consent document and the principal risk would be potential harm resulting from a breach of confidentiality. Each subject will be asked whether the subject wants documentation linking the subject with the research, and the subject's wishes will govern.

- The research presents no more than minimal risk of harm to subjects and involves no procedures for which written consent is normally required outside of the research context.

In cases in which the documentation requirement is waived, the IRB may require the investigator to provide subjects with a written statement regarding the research.

EXCULPATORY LANGUAGE IN THE CONSENT DOCUMENT

MICHELE RUSSELL-EINHORN, THOMAS PUGLISI, AND ROBERT J. AMDUR

Exculpatory Language in the Consent Document

The IRB should consider *exculpatory language* to be any language "through which the subject or the representative is made to waive or appear to waive *any* of the subject's legal rights." Thus, any language waiving or appearing to waive any legal right (regardless of the nature of that right) is prohibited.

- The following statements are examples of exculpatory language:

  1. I agree that the medical center will not pay me for any injuries that I might sustain as a result of participating in this research.

  2. I understand that the institution will not share with me any profits received from the sale or commercialization of any cells developed in this research.

  3. I agree that everything in this consent form is adequate and complies with the regulations.

  4. I understand that I will not sue the sponsor or the investigator for any negligence.

  5. Subjects agree to hold harmless all institutions, investigators, or sponsors affiliated with or in any way a part of this research protocol.

Investigators are frequently admonished by their IRBs to refrain from using exculpatory language in their informed consent documents. Almost as frequently, this admonishment comes with little or no explanation of what constitutes "exculpatory language." Indeed, many IRBs seem confused about where to draw the line in determining whether a proposed statement is exculpatory. Here is what federal regulations say about exculpatory language in the consent process:

> No informed consent, whether oral or written, may include any exculpatory language through which the subject is made to waive or appear to waive any of the subject's legal rights, or releases or appears to release the investigator, the sponsor, the institution, or its agents from liability for negligence.

THE NARROW (BUT "INCORRECT") INTERPRETATION

A narrow interpretation of the regulatory language would limit the prohibition to statements involving a release from liability for negligence. Those who argue in favor of the narrow interpretation point out that in common usage (as verified by any current dictionary), the word *exculpatory* relates to lack of guilt. This is also the case relative to its usage in law. According to *Black's Law Dictionary*, the word involves clearing "from alleged fault or guilt" or releasing "from liability" for "wrongful acts."

THE BROAD ("CORRECT") INTERPRETATION

These arguments notwithstanding, the federal agencies that regulate research have a long history of applying a much broader interpretation of the exculpatory language prohibition. A careful reading of the regulatory language reveals that, in this context, the meaning of the phrase *exculpatory language* is expanded to include any language "through which the subject or the representative is made to waive or appear to waive *any* of the subject's legal rights." Thus any language waiving or appearing to waive any legal right (regardless of the nature of that right) is prohibited.

PRACTICAL APPLICATIONS

In a practical sense, exculpatory statements tend to be statements in which a subject in a research protocol is asked to agree to or accept something, usually something unfavorable to the subject. A statement that sets forth simple facts, on the other hand, is usually not likely to be viewed as exculpatory.

Examples of Language That Is *Not* Exculpatory

In the following examples, the institution simply sets forth the facts describing the institution's intent and policy. These statements would not be considered exculpatory under the regulations and would be permissible.

1. The University Medical School has no policy or plan to pay for any injuries you might receive as a result of participating in this research protocol.

2. Tissue obtained from you in this research may be used to establish a cell line that could be patented and licensed. There are no plans to provide financial compensation to you should this occur.

3. By consenting to participate, you authorize the use of your bodily fluids and tissue samples for the research described above.

Examples of Exculpatory Language

1. I agree that the medical center will not pay me for any injuries that I might sustain as a result of participating in this research.

2. I understand that the institution will not share with me any profits received from the sale or commercialization of any cells developed in this research.

3. I agree that everything in this consent form is adequate and complies with the regulations.

4. I understand that I will not sue the sponsor or the investigator for any negligence.

5. Subjects agree to hold harmless all institutions, investigators, or sponsors affiliated with or in any way a part of this research protocol.

Again, a good rule of thumb is to state simply the factual situation and avoid any statement that requires the agreement or concurrence of the subject.

EXCLUDING (POTENTIALLY) PREGNANT WOMEN FROM RESEARCH

BRUCE G. GORDON, ERNEST D. PRENTICE, AND
ROBERT J. AMDUR

Evaluating a Study That Excludes Pregnant or Potentially Pregnant Women

- There are three arguments that support the exclusion of pregnant women:

  1. Nonmaleficence (do no harm, minimize risk)

  2. Improve scientific quality

  3. Decrease the chance of a lawsuit for the investigator or sponsor

- The argument to include pregnant women is based on an interpretation of the Belmont principle of justice, which says that the risks and potential benefits of research participation should be distributed equitably among the types of people who are likely to benefit from the research results.

- An attempt to exclude women of childbearing potential from research participation is based on the concept that if it is ethical to exclude women who are known to be pregnant then it is ethical to exclude all women who could become pregnant during the course of the study.

- The IRB should not approve a study that excludes women of childbearing potential from research participation based on the risk to a fetus.

This chapter presents guidelines for evaluating the ethics of a general policy to exclude women from research because of concern about the risk of study participation to a fetus. The issues involved with research in which pregnant women or fetuses are the primary subject of research are discussed in other chapters in this handbook.

There are three situations where IRB members will encounter the "exclusion because of pregnancy" issue: (1) The exclusion of pregnant women, (2) the exclusion of women of childbearing potential, and (3) the requirement for birth control. In order to analyze this aspect of study design, it is important for IRB members to understand the arguments for and against routinely excluding pregnant women from research participation when the risk to the fetus is significant or unknown.

THE PRINCIPLES OF NONMALEFICENCE AND JUSTICE

The main ethical argument for excluding pregnant women from research where there is even a remote chance of harm to the fetus is the principle of "non-maleficence," which means that research should be conducted in a manner that does not cause harm. This concept is reflected in item 6 of the Nuremberg Code: "No experiment should be conducted where there is an a priori reason to believe that death or disabling injury will occur." It is also seen in federal regulations where a requirement for IRB approval of research is a study design that "minimizes risks to subjects."

Two related arguments for excluding pregnant women from research participation are scientific quality and the risk of personal injury lawsuit for the investigator or sponsor. The scientific quality argument says that pregnant women are likely to respond differently to study interventions than other subjects such that their inclusion will compromise the persuasiveness of research results. The lawsuit liability argument is straightforward to understand. Although it is beyond the scope of this book to discuss either of these arguments in detail, we can summarize them by saying that these factors have played a minor role in directed the thinking of the regulatory and ethics community on the question of excluding pregnant women from research when the woman is the primary research subject and there might be risk to a fetus. As described below, the scientific quality argument is directly contradicted by the main argument in favor including pregnant women in research in most settings. The lawsuit issue may be important from the standpoint of a study sponsor but it is a peripheral issue for the IRB.

The main argument in favor of including pregnant women in most research activities is that to not do so violates the Belmont principle of justice as discussed in Chapter 1-4 of this handbook. Basically, the principle of justice requires that "the potential risk and benefits of research should be distributed equally among those who may benefit from the research." If research participation may directly benefit the subject, then denying a pregnant woman the right to make the decision about research participation is viewed as paternalistic to an unacceptable degree. When research is primarily designed to benefit future members of society, the rationale for including pregnant women is that research results are usually applied to all members of society—including pregnant women.

It may be useful for IRB members to understand how federal regulations have changed over the past twenty-five years in response to the debate about routinely excluding women who are, or could become, pregnant from participating in research where the risk to the fetus is significant or unknown. The regulatory history of this issue is described in detail in *Institutional Review Board: Management and Function*, the textbook discussed in Chapter 1-1. Basically the story is this:

- In the mid-1970s, several federal agencies, including the Food and Drug Administration (FDA), established regulations that supported the policy that pregnant women, and women who could become pregnant, should be excluded from most studies that involved investigational medications.

- In mid-1984, a federal task force expressed the opinion that a long-standing lack of research in women's health had compromised the quality of available information on diseases affecting women.

- In 1993, the FDA issued "Guideline for Study and Evaluation of Gender Differences in the Clinical Evaluation of Drugs." This articulated the agency's decision to reverse the 1977 policy that had barred most women from participating in the early phases of clinical trials.

- In 1994, the National Institutes of Health (NIH) issued "Guidelines on Inclusion of Women and Minorities as Subjects in Clinical Research," which stated that "women ... must be included in all NIH-supported biomedical and behavioral research projects involving human subjects unless a clear and compelling rationale and justification establishes ... that inclusion is inappropriate."

- In 1998, the Department of Health and Human Services (DHHS) issued a proposed amendment to the research regulations. Among the many changes, the proposed change "institutes a policy of presumed opportunity for inclusion of pregnant women in research." The amendment was approved by DHHS Secretary Donna Shalala, but subsequent enactment was delayed by President Bush.

EXCLUDING WOMEN OF CHILDBEARING POTENTIAL

It is important to understand that the ethics of excluding women who have the potential to become pregnant during a study—sometimes referred to as "women of childbearing potential"—is simply a variation on the debate about including women who are known to be pregnant. The concept is that if it is ethical to exclude pregnant women because of risk to the fetus then it is ethical to exclude all women of childbearing potential because it is not possible to eliminate the chance that pregnancy will develop during the course of the study.

As described above, federal regulations have been revised over the past decade to reflect a change in how our society thinks about the rights of women to make decisions about research participation. Basically, the current thinking is that it is unethical to exclude women of childbearing potential from participating in research based on concern about the risk to the fetus that would exist if a woman became pregnant during the course of the study. In other words, the risks of research participation to the state of pregnancy are risks that women in general should be given the right to make a decision about. It is perfectly acceptable to exclude individuals from research participation if they are not capable of understanding the risks of research participation, or to exclude individuals who do not intend to comply with a research requirement, but it is not acceptable to exclude a general class of women based on the capacity for pregnancy.

REQUIRING THE USE OF BIRTH CONTROL

The requirement that women of childbearing potential use birth control during research participation represents a compromise between the competing desires to exclude pregnant women and to include women of childbearing potential who are not pregnant. By making the use of birth control a requirement for research participation, the investigator is attempting to decrease the chance of pregnancy as much as possible. In many studies, the IRB will determine that a requirement for contraception is essential to minimize the risk of research participation. However, it is important for IRB members to understand that requiring birth control does not mean that it is acceptable to exclude women who are known to be pregnant. These are separate issues that require separate determinations by the IRB based on the principles discussed above.

Bioethicists, federal authorities, and IRB members will likely debate the inclusion of pregnant women in research for decades to come. At this time, it is not possible to present a blanket directive for how the IRB should vote on any given situation. When a study proposes to exclude women because they are, or may become pregnant, IRB members should understand that they should make a determination based on their evaluation of a tradeoff between the principles of nonmaleficence and justice.

BANKING OF BIOLOGIC TISSUES FOR RESEARCH

KAREN M. HANSEN, ROBERT J. AMDUR, AND ELIZABETH A. BANKERT

Template Consent Document Wording to Bank Tissue for Research

The following template wording should be used in the consent document to request permission to bank (store) tissue for a well-defined and explicitly described set of tests in the future:

- We ask your permission to test your blood or tissue for research.

- Will you be given the results of research tests?

The following template wording should be used in the consent document to request permission to bank (store) tissue when the exact tests that may be done on the tissue in the future *cannot* be described at this time:

- We are asking you to donate your blood or tissue for future research.

- Will the blood or tissue that you donate be tested for diseases?

- Will you or your doctor be given research results?

- What research studies will be done on the blood or tissue that you donate?

- Will you be paid for donating blood or tissue for future research?

- Are there risks to donating your blood or tissue for future research?

The IRB is likely to encounter two different scenarios that involve a request to collect or store a person's blood or tissue for research. An important difference between the two scenarios emerges if the investigator can explain exactly which tests will be done on the tissue at the time that informed consent is initially requested to bank the tissue. In many cases, requests to bank tissue for research are presented as a secondary part of another study. Template wording in the consent document for the request to bank tissue will improve the chance that subjects have the information they need to make an informed decision and help focus IRB members on the issues that are important to evaluate with this category of research.

TEMPLATE WORDING

The consent document should say the following when requesting permission to bank (store) tissue for a well-defined and explicitly described set of tests in the future:

- **We ask your permission to test your blood or tissue for research.** This study includes laboratory tests that will analyze samples of your blood or tissues. [If additional procedures, such as blood draws or biopsies, will be needed for this study, describe them here, including risks.] Blood or tissue samples will be sent to a laboratory where tests will be performed. The purpose of the tests that will be done on your blood or tissue is to determine … [complete this sentence].

- **Will you be given the results of research tests?** The results from these tests will not be sent to you or your doctor, and will not be used in planning your care. You will not be able to find out the results of these tests even if you ask for them. These tests are only for research purposes. [If this not the case, explain the conditions under which subjects or their physicians will have access to these results. If the subject or their physician will have access to test results, you must explain the potential risks and implications of this disclosure. When applicable, discuss the need for genetic or psychological counseling before or after the study.]

- **Do you give us permission to test your blood or tissue?** Please indicate if you agree to participate by circling your "Yes" or "No" response below. You do not have to give permission to use your blood or tissue for research to participate in the other parts of this study. If you do not want your blood or tissue to be tested in this part of the study, it will not affect your care at this institution or the ability to receive treatment as part of this study. Please ask questions if you do not understand why we are asking for your permission to use your blood or tissue for research or if you would like more information about any part of this study.

  I agree to participate in the part of the study that involves testing of my blood or tissue as described above. Please circle YES or NO and sign your name below.

The consent document should say the following when requesting permission to bank (store) tissue when the exact tests that may be done on the tissue in the future cannot be described at the time that informed consent is initially obtained:

- **We are asking you to donate your blood or tissue for future research.** We are requesting your permission to donate some of your blood or tissue for future research. The blood or tissue samples that will be stored are left over from specimens that were taken, or will be taken, as part of your routine medical care [or as part of this study (if the tissue banking request is an add-on study within a primary study)]. [If additional procedures, such as blood draws or biopsies, will be done to procure the specimens that will be stored, this must be explained along with any associated risks.]

- **Will the blood or tissue that you donate be tested for diseases?** Some people are worried about their blood or tissue being tested for things that indicate that they have a particular disease or problem, or that a disease or problem is in the genes of your family—for example, a test for AIDS or for the gene that indicates Huntington's chorea.

  At this time there is no plan to test your blood or tissue for things that indicate that you or your biologic relatives have a serious disease or problem. [If this is not the case then describe the relevant tests and the potential implications and risks. When applicable, discuss the need for genetic or psychological counseling before or after the study.]

- **Will you or your doctor be given research results?** It is very important that you understand that the results from tests that are done on the blood or tissue that you donate for future research will not be given to you or your doctor, even if you ask that this be done. Any such results will not be sent to your hospital medical record. These tests will be done only for research purposes. [If subjects or their physician will have access to research results, describe the circumstances of this access and the potential implications and risks. When applicable, discuss the need for genetic or psychological counseling before or after the study.]

- **What research studies will be done on the blood or tissue that you donate?** At this time, it is impossible to name all of the kinds of studies that researchers may want to use your blood or tissue for. Any research done on your blood or tissue in the future must be approved by a committee called an Institutional Review Board that is set up to determine that the research is done according to accepted standards.

- **Will the blood or tissue that you donate be sold in the future?** Your blood or tissue will be used only for research and will not be sold.

- **Will you be paid for donating blood or tissue for future research?** No. You will not be paid for the blood or tissue that you are now being asked to donate for future research. Although it is possible that future research done on your blood and tissue may help to develop something that is commercially valuable—something that makes a lot of money for somebody—you will not receive payment for any commercial activity that results from research with your blood or tissues.

- **Will you be penalized if you decide not to donate blood or tissue for research?** No. You will not be penalized in any way for not donating blood or tissue for future research. If you decide not to donate blood or tissue for future research, it will not affect your medical care [or your ability to participate in the treatment part of this study (if tissue storage is being requested as an add-on study within a primary study)].

- **Why would you donate your blood or tissue for future research?** Because research with your blood or tissue may lead to discoveries that will help people in the future.

- **Are there risks to donating your blood or tissue for future research?** Donating your blood or tissue for future research may have no risk. However, a serious risk that should be considered is the possibility that someone will learn things about you that you don't want them to know. It is difficult to estimate if this is a possibility in your case because we don't know exactly what studies may be done on your blood or tissue in the future. However, all reasonable efforts will be made to protect the confidentiality of infor- mation that can in any way be connected to you. As in many other kinds of research, certain authorities do have the right to review your research file. In addition to research directors, the people that may have access to your research information are representatives from the U.S. Food and Drug Administration as well as the Institutional Review Board, a committee that is set up to determine that research is done according to accepted standards.

- **Do you have any additional questions?**

    If you have questions about your rights as a research participant, please call ...

    If you have questions about specimen and/or data storage, please call ...

    If you have questions about your medical treatment or emergency care, please call ...

- **Making your choice.** Please put an X in the boxes below to indicate if you want to donate your blood or tissue for future research.

☐ Yes, I will donate my blood or tissue for future research. Please also check one of the following boxes:

    ☐ There are no restrictions on the kind of research that may be done with my blood or tissue:

OR

    ☐ You may use my blood or tissue for future research as long as the only kind of research that is done is research to improve the understanding or treatment of [name specific diseases or conditions].

☐ No, I do not want to donate my blood or tissue for future research.

Please sign your name here: _____

CHAPTER 3-13

PLACEBO-CONTROLLED TRIALS

ROBERT J. AMDUR

Evaluating the Ethics of a Placebo-Controlled Trial

Decision points in the algorithm for evaluating the ethics of a placebo-controlled trial are as follows:

- Is placebo used in place of or in addition to standard therapy?

- Is standard therapy considered to be effective?

- Is the toxicity of standard therapy such that patients routinely refuse treatment?

- Could the use of a placebo in place of standard therapy cause irreversible health problems or severe suffering?

- Is it possible to estimate the placebo response rate in this study with a reasonable degree of accuracy?

- Evaluate the credibility of altruism using the reasonable-person standard: Could this trial benefit future patients to the point that a reasonable-person with an average degree of altruism and risk-aversiveness would consent to being randomized in this trial?

The use of a placebo in clinical research studies is currently a topic of active debate in the medical literature. At one end of the spectrum is the argument that the current use of a placebo is often unethical because alternate study designs would produce results that are of similar value to society with less risk to individual research participants. The counterargument is that current policy regarding the use of placebos is essential to protect society from the harm that would result from the widespread use of ineffective medical treatments. A decision algorithm that will help IRB members evaluate the ethics of a clinical research trial that involves concomitant placebo control is shown as Figure 3.1.

THE USE OF PLACEBO IN PLACE OF STANDARD THERAPY

The first step in evaluating the ethics of a placebo-controlled trial is to decide if a placebo is being used in place of standard therapy. Standard therapy may be a type of active treatment (for example, a medication with treatment-specific activity); supportive care, meaning treatment designed to alleviate symptoms but without specific activity for the underlying medical condition; or no treatment. From the ethical standpoint, the potential problem with placebo therapy is that it exposes patients to a treatment that has no specific activity for their disease. When an available therapy is considered to be beneficial, the use of a placebo *instead of* accepted therapy may be unethical. However, when a placebo is being used *in addition* to standard therapy, as is done in add-on and sequential treatment study designs, there is no ethical tension related to the use of treatment without disease-specific activity.

The Efficacy of Standard Therapy

The second decision point is to determine if standard therapy is considered to be effective. With medical conditions where there are no good treatment options, there may be legitimate controversy about the value of standard therapy. When standard therapy does not meaningfully improve length or quality of life, it is ethical to enroll informed subjects in research that uses a placebo in

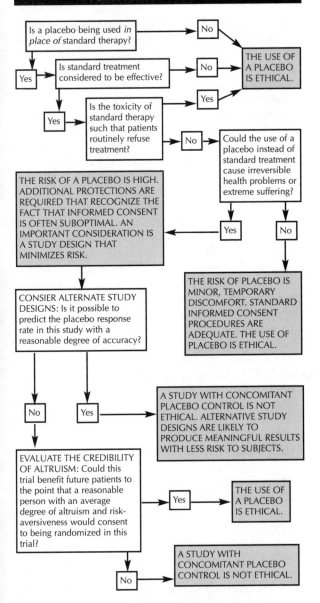

Figure 3.1 From Robert J. Amdur and C.J. Biddle, "An Algorithm for Evaluating the Ethics of a Placebo-Controlled Trial," *Int. J. Cancer (Radiat. Oncol. Invest)* 96 (2001): 261–269.

place of standard treatment. However, when standard therapy is considered to be effective in the study population, additional issues must be evaluated to determine if it is ethical to use a placebo in place of standard therapy.

Evaluating the efficacy of standard therapy may not be straightforward because controversy often exists regarding the treatment-specific activity of approaches that are commonly recommended. In the absence of overwhelming evidence, some experts will question the efficacy of treatment that is considered to be beneficial by other segments of the medical community. From an ethical standpoint, a lack of consensus within the overall medical community is less important than the opinion of the local physicians who will be asking patients to participate in research. The practice of medicine is based on the judgment of individual physicians taking care of specific patients. The evidence that a given medical treatment will or will not be effective in a specific patient is often not definitive. For this reason, the ethics of a placebo in a given community is best evaluated by asking local physicians how they would manage a patient who decides not to participate in research. At this point in the decision algorithm, the critical question is whether physicians who will be asking patients to participate in the study think that standard therapy is beneficial to the point that they routinely recommend it to their patients.

THE TOXICITY OF STANDARD TREATMENT

The potential problem with the use of a placebo in medical research is that subjects will be denied beneficial treatment. When evaluating the potential benefit of a medical treatment, it is important to consider both efficacy and toxicity. If the toxicity of available treatments is such that patients routinely refuse therapy that is known to have direct activity against their disease process, then it is ethical to conduct research that treats informed subjects with placebo in place of standard therapy. However, when standard treatment is both effective and well tolerated, other factors must be evaluated to determine the ethics of a placebo-controlled medical research trial.

As with treatment efficacy, there may be disagreement within the medical community about the level of toxicity of a given medical treatment in a specific patient population. Opinions about the overall effect of medical treatment are appropriately influenced to a large degree by personal values and individual experience. As discussed above, the important question from an ethical standpoint is how the physicians who will be enrolling subjects in research view the risk/benefit profile of standard therapy. Again, the way a physician manages patients outside the setting of a research protocol usually indicates that physician's opinion about the value of alternative therapies.

TEMPORARY DISCOMFORT VERSUS IRREVERSIBLE HARM

Much of the recent literature on ethical requirements for the use of placebos has emphasized the importance of making a distinction between the use of a placebo in a setting that increases the risk of temporary discomfort and use of a placebo in a way that increases the risk of severe morbidity or irreversible health problems. This distinction is not discussed in federal research regulations or in ethical guidelines such as the Nuremberg Code, Declaration of Helsinki, and Belmont Report. The basic concept is that protections that recognize the inherent vulnerability of medical research subjects and the limitations of the informed consent process are needed when the risk associated with placebo treatment is high. In practical terms, this means that the fact that a subject enrolls in a study following a process that complies with the standard requirements for informed consent does not mean that the study is ethical.

Concern about the quality and circumstances of informed consent is not unique to research that involves placebos. An extensive body of literature now supports the view that in many medical situations it is not possible to obtain the type of informed consent that is considered to be a requirement for ethical research. When the risk of research participation is high, any imperfection in the consent process has a major effect on research ethics. When the use of placebo carries a risk of irreversible and serious harm, the ethics of research will hinge on the ability of alternate study designs to provide valuable information on the study question with less risk to research subjects.

At the other extreme is the situation where the risk of placebo is limited to minor, temporary discomfort. In this setting it is appropriate that research standards rely on the informed consent process to create an environment where subjects understand the main implications of their decision to participate in research and important decisions are made without coercion.

CONSIDERING ALTERNATIVE STUDY DESIGNS

A fundamental ethical standard is that research should be designed so that the risks to subjects are minimized and reasonable in relation to anticipated benefits. A major element of the placebo controversy is debate over the implications of using alternative study designs to evaluate the efficacy of new medical treatments. This is a complex topic without definitive answers to several important questions.

As a society, we want to design clinical trials to minimize the chance of a false-positive result. The scientific quality of a clinical trial refers to the aspects of the study that influence the credibility and persuasiveness of research results. The relationship between study quality and the use of concomitant placebo control is a complex and controversial topic. The main issue is the value of a positive result in a trial with placebo versus active control. A point/counterpoint approach is used to explain the different schools of thought on this subject:

The Value of a Positive Result in a Trial with Concomitant Placebo Versus Active Control

Point

Scientific quality is superior with a study design that involves concomitant placebo control because it is usually not possible to accurately determine important statistical parameters in a trial that compares a study treatment with an active control. This is especially true in medical conditions where variability in the placebo response rate is known to be high.

The fundamental question is different in a trial with active control than in a trial with placebo control. Trials that randomize subjects between study treatment and placebos use a study design that directly evaluates efficacy. Trials that use active treatment control are classified as *noninferiority trials* because the goal is to show that the study drug is not less effective than the control by more than a defined amount. A fundamental assumption of a noninferiority trial with active control is that noninferiority is evidence of equivalence.

A major argument against using a noninferiority (equivalence) trial to make conclusions about treatment efficacy is that there is no accepted way to estimate some of the important statistical parameters needed to minimize the chance of a false-positive result. The main problem is that a noninferiority trial requires an estimate of a parameter called the *noninferiority margin*, which describes the degree of inferiority of the study medication (compared with active control) that the trial will attempt to exclude statistically. The value of the noninferiority margin is usually based on past experience in placebo-controlled trials, but clinical judgment also plays a role.

Estimating the noninferiority margin is especially difficult when there is variability in the placebo response rate between trials. For this reason, support for trials with concomitant placebo control is generally strongest in medical conditions where variability in the placebo response rate is likely to be large. There are many medical conditions for which medications that are considered to be effective cannot regularly be shown to be superior to placebo in well-designed clinical trials.

Uncertainty in the design of a clinical trial compromises the credibility of study results. Lack of confidence in the scientific quality of an active-control trial is such that much of the scientific community, including some FDA officials, view a noninferiority trial using active control as a crude tool for evaluating the efficacy of unproven therapy in a wide range of medical conditions. People with this point of view argue that trials with concurrent placebo control are essential to protect society from the harm that will result from approving new medical therapies based on false-positive results from noninferiority studies.

Counterpoint

This is an example of a situation where many of the experts are mistaken. The scientific quality of results from placebo-controlled trials is overrated. The value of results from a noninferiority trial with active control is often underrated. Society would not be worse off if the FDA approval of new medical treatments were based on the results of noninferiority trials with comparison to standard therapy (concomitant active control) in many of the situations where concomitant placebo control is currently required.

Arguments that support the use of placebo control in ethically controversial situations frequently include dogmatic statements about placebo-controlled trials being the "gold standard" for evaluating the efficacy of new medical treatments. These positions imply that a placebo-controlled trial is unquestionably the most accurate way to evaluate treatment efficacy. Critics argue that there is no convincing evidence to support this concept. For example, in a recent review of studies used to support FDA approval of antidepressant medications—a prime example of a situation where experts argue that the large variability in placebo response rate demands the use of placebo control—the author concluded, "We can see from the data presented that standard therapy is almost always superior to placebo and similar in effectiveness to the investigational drugs that later gained market approval. Thus therapeutic equivalence trials would have led to the same conclusions regarding effectiveness of the investigational medications as placebo-controlled trials. So why withhold effective treatment that is likely to benefit patients?" (Michels, K. B., *Arch Gen Psychiatry* 2000, 57: 321–322). In a 1994 article in the *New England Journal of Medicine*, Rothman and Michels commented on statements about the superiority of placebo control that are frequently found in FDA documents and research textbooks: "Without justification, such statements confer on placebo control a stature that ranks it with double blinding and randomization as a hallmark of good science…. No scientific principle, however, requires the comparison in a trial to involve a placebo instead of, or in addition to, an active treatment" (*NEJM* 331 [1994]: 394–397).

EVALUATING THE CREDIBILITY OF ALTRUISM USING THE REASONABLE-PERSON STANDARD

Probably the most controversial aspect of the placebo debate concerns the tradeoff between the welfare of the individuals who will be the subjects of research and the welfare of people in the future who may benefit from research results. Obviously, this tension exists in other areas of research, but the importance of the "individual versus society" issue to the placebo debate cannot be overemphasized. In a biomedical research study where the use of placebo increases the risk of irreversible harm, the only way to justify the use of placebo is to argue that it is ethical to increase risk to current subjects to produce information that may benefit people in the future. A major problem with this argument is that most guidelines related to research ethics stress the importance of not sacrificing the individual for the sake of society in general or future subjects. Clearly there are situations where the trade-off between individual welfare and societal benefit is acceptable, but each person who is asked to make a determination on this issue in a specific study must decide what is acceptable and unacceptable based on personal values.

There is no question that altruism may be an acceptable reason for a person to participate in research, regardless of the potential for increased risk. However, to accept the altruism argument, one must assume full and voluntary informed consent. When considering this argument, it is important to understand that an extensive body of literature now exists supporting the view that, in many medical situations, the researcher cannot obtain the type of informed consent considered to be a requirement for ethical research. The documentation of informed consent is not credible when the nature of the study is such that reasonable people would not volunteer to participate in the research if they had a clear understanding of the implications of their decision.

No definitive formula can be used to determine when a trade-off between the welfare of individual subjects and future patients is acceptable. A bioethicist named Baruch Brody has discussed a "reasonable person" standard for evaluating the ethics of clinical trials. In the context of the placebo discussion, the reasonable-person standard says that a randomized, placebo-controlled trial is justified only if (1) the subjects have validly consented to being randomized, and (2) a reasonable person of an average degree of altruism and risk-aversiveness might consent to being randomized. This reasonable-person standard articulates the criteria that should be used to evaluate the ethics of placebo in the final decision point of the placebo algorithm.

TREATMENT WITHHOLDING AND WASHOUT PERIODS

RICHARD FERRELL AND ROBERT J. AMDUR

Treatment Withholding and Washout Periods

The criteria that apply for IRB approval of research involving a placebo are equally relevant to research involving withholding of active treatment.

- The IRB should use the placebo-controlled algorithm presented in the chapter dealing with placebo-controlled trials to evaluate the ethics of trials that withhold treatment in psychiatric research.

- The main issues to consider when evaluating a study that withholds active treatment for a period of time are the potential for severe suffering or permanent disability, the value of standard therapy in the study population, and rescue plans.

- When evaluating a study that withholds active treatment in patients with schizophrenia, the IRB should consider making voluntary hospitalization or very close and careful outpatient care during the period of highest risk a requirement for IRB approval.

This chapter will focus on the specific class of psychiatric drug studies in which active treatment is withheld for a period of time that may have an important effect on disease status. There is overlap between the issues of treatment withdrawal and placebo control because in both situations there is a period of time when participants receive no active therapy. The bottom line is that, from the standpoint of IRB evaluations, a treatment withholding or washout period is simply a version of the placebo control issue. For this reason, IRB members should use the algorithm dealing with placebo-controlled trials presented in Chapter 3-13 to evaluate the ethics of studies that require the withholding of active treatment.

A SELECTIVE LITERATURE REVIEW

The National Alliance for the Mentally Ill (NAMI) has published standards designed to protect the welfare of psychiatric research participants. Although NAMI has taken no official position on treatment withholding, prominent advocates from this organization have expressed concern about studies that do so:

> Many NAMI members now feel that a placebo is not acceptable, because we view schizophrenia and other psychotic disorders and affective illness as life-threatening diseases…. Indeed, NAMI has serious questions about whether placebo-controlled studies are still necessary in this era. Researchers conducting such studies must be incredibly vigilant about these issues in their informed consent process, ongoing communication with families and patients, and follow-up to the research.

Several experts in the treatment of schizophrenia have seriously questioned the ethics of "washout" studies in schizophrenia. For example, at the thirty-third annual NAMI meeting in San Juan, Puerto Rico, Dr. Haas argued that delayed treatment of schizophrenia causes negative long-term effects. It is indeed hard to imagine how one could argue that delaying treatment could benefit a sick individual, unless one maintains that treatment is more likely to do harm than good.

GUIDELINES FOR IRB REVIEW

It is important to recognize that the criteria that apply for IRB approval of research involving a placebo are equally relevant to research involving the withholding of active treatment. The IRB should use the placebo-controlled algorithm presented in Chapter 3-13 to evaluate the ethics of trials that withhold treatment in psychiatric research. The main issues to consider are the nature of the patient's condition, the value of standard therapy in the study population, and rescue plans.

This chapter will not repeat the criteria explained in Chapter 3-13. When making a decision about approving a protocol, IRB members should not hesitate to ask for the opinion of an unbiased expert regarding the questions that the IRB needs to answer. Also, when evaluating a study that withholds active treatment in patients with schizophrenia, the IRB should consider making voluntary hospitalization or very close and careful outpatient care during the period of highest risk a requirement for IRB approval.

CASE DISCUSSIONS

Example 1

A proposed study will compare two dosage schedules of an investigational antipsychotic drug for the treatment of schizophrenia. Previous studies with this drug over the dose range in this study suggest a favorable risk/benefit profile. Subjects whose symptoms are not optimally controlled on standard medications will have a seven-day washout period during which they receive no medication. The clinician investigator has the option of reducing this period to three days depending upon clinical judgment about the participant's condition. The study requires close monitoring of participants throughout the study with plans for immediate rescue treatment and/or hospitalization if symptoms worsen.

Withholding treatment is ethical in this study primarily because the period without treatment is brief and flexible depending on the severity of the illness. Symptom control was suboptimal on standard therapy, and the study provides for close monitoring with appropriate rescue. The IRB should approve the study.

Example 2

A study will investigate treatment of attention-deficit/hyperactivity disorder (ADHD) in children with a new long-acting formulation of methylphenidate (Ritalin) that is taken only once a day. An inclusion criterion is that patients are currently well controlled on the standard form of methylphenidate, which is given multiple times per day. The study requires a two-week washout period when all subjects will be given a placebo. Subjects who do well on the placebo (minimal symptoms of ADHD) are excluded from the remainder of the study. Subjects who deteriorate on the placebo are then randomized to treatment with the new formulation of methylphenidate or placebo for a four-week study period.

The purpose of the washout period in this study is to identify subjects who are benefiting from methylphenidate treatment. The study is designed with a goal of producing symptom deterioration in a subgroup of study subjects. Consultation with several people who had experience with uncontrolled ADHD children in the classroom stressed that even a few weeks of symptom deterioration may be a serious problem for the child with ADHD and other children in the classroom. The Dartmouth IRB did not approve a study similar to this.

PHASE I ONCOLOGY TRIALS

MATHEW MILLER AND ROBERT J. AMDUR

Phase I Oncology Trials

Phase 1 oncology trials are designed to produce significant toxicity with no planned direct benefit to research subjects.

- "Therapeutic misconception" explains why people participate in Phase 1 oncology trials—meaning that they falsely believe that the study is designed out of concern for their well-being.

- Require standardized wording in the consent document as follows:

Purpose: The purpose of this study is to find the highest dose of _____ that people can tolerate without getting extremely ill.

Risks: In this study, the dose of _____ will be increased until people get extremely sick. It is impossible to predict the side effects that you will experience.

Benefits: This study is not being done to treat your cancer. Based on prior experience, the chance that you will feel better or live longer as a result of participating in this study is almost zero. This study is being done in the hope that it will provide information that will improve the treatment of people in the future.

A fundamental tension in human experimentation on patients arises from the inherent conflict between the goals of science and those of clinical care. Phase I cancer trials embody this conflict in perhaps its purest and most intensified form because the subjects in these trials are terminally ill patients and the scientific goal is to effect toxicity—not cure, remission, or palliation. This presents special challenges to IRB review, especially in light of empirical evidence that patients overwhelmingly enroll in these trials seeking physical benefit. The bioethicist Benjamin Freedman summarized the fundamental issue:

> A Phase 1 study of drug X is often said to be a study of X's safety and efficacy. Calling a toxicity study a study of safety seems harmless, and perhaps even reflects a laudably optimistic view of the world. Calling it a study of efficacy is, however, simply false; although to be sure, were there no hope of this drug's working it would not be tested.

BACKGROUND

In the course of developing new anticancer compounds, agents that have demonstrated promise in cell culture and animal models must at some time be tested in human subjects. In these initial or *Phase 1* human trials, compounds are administered to terminally ill cancer patients in an attempt to estimate the highest dose human beings can tolerate. Evaluating a drug's anti-cancer effect in human cancers, a primary objective of subsequent Phase 2 and Phase 3 trials, is not a defined goal in Phase 1 studies.

Phase 1 dose-toxicity information is usually gathered by administering increasing doses of a new drug (or of novel combinations of known agents) to successive cohorts of three to six patients. Once serious but reversible toxic effects are produced in a fixed proportion of patients (often one-third of the patients in the highest-dose cohort) the trial ends. Since most responses occur at 80 to 120 percent of the maximum tolerated dose, subjects enrolled in the earliest cohorts have the least risk of severe toxicity but also the least likelihood of a clinical response. Thus the predominant cohort-specific dose escalation schemes are at odds with what patients generally assume about the primacy of their interests—for example, that each patient will receive a dose that attempts to maximize the chance for anticancer effect.

PLANNED TOXICITY AND NO DIRECT BENEFIT

The predominant structure of Phase 1 trials embodies peculiarly contrasting tensions at opposing ends of the dosing spectrum. At one extreme, requiring that at least one patient suffer severe (but reversible) toxicity; at the other, subjecting 60 to 80 percent of patients to doses that, based on preclinical models, are *a priori* expected to prove less likely to produce a response than higher achievable levels. Given a remission rate of under 1 percent in Phase 1 trials, and a comparable rate of death due to drug toxicity, few would claim any aggregate survival advantage for participants.

THERAPEUTIC MISCONCEPTIONS OF SUBJECTS

There is now a large body of evidence recognizing the process of "therapeutic misconception"—a misunderstanding whereby patients do not fully recognize the way that science sometimes deprives them of care chosen solely out of concern for their well-being. Phase 1 cancer patients thus agree to participate in these trials largely in hope of physical benefit and generally assume that the structure of the trial itself serves their personal therapeutic goal (see Chapter 10-13 in *Institutional Review Board: Management and Function* for a detailed discussion of these data).

RECOMMENDATIONS FOR THE IRB

1. **Determine if the study agent is being evaluated simultaneously in other centers.** Phase 1 research studies that seek to repeat other Phase 1 trials or are contemporaneous with others trials of the same agent must justify the rationale for repetition and must demonstrate, in the case of contemporaneous trials, how the centers will coordinate their dosing strategies based on the daily exchange of shared data. As the bioethicist Jay Katz has written, "we must not seek truth when it is already known or progress when it is already a reality."

2. **Reject justifications for a Phase 1 protocol that are based on adjunctive elements unrelated to the research question.** Arguments that the general quality of the medical care that they receive will be higher if they participate in a research study should never offset ethical compromises in research design. Subjects should not participate in a Phase 1 trial because they benefit from "close follow-up" or have access to "free medical care."

3. **Make clear the distinction between research and patient care.** IRBs should reject in all written forms and should discourage, in the consenting dialogue itself, the use of oxymoronic language that serves to blur the distinction between the enterprise of research and the activity of patient-centered care.

4. **Require a commitment to eliminating misconceptions about risks and benefits.**

The Belmont principle of respect for persons emphasizes the need to clarify the goals of Phase 1 trials to the people who are being asked to participate in them. Specifically, potential subjects should be told that Phase 1 trials are designed to determine toxicity, that severe toxicity is a planned event for a subset of subjects, and that direct benefit is both not intended and extremely unlikely.

5. **Require standardized wording in the consent document as follows:**

Purpose: The purpose of this study is to find the highest dose of _____ that people can tolerate without getting extremely ill.

Risks: In this study, the dose of _____will be increased until people get extremely sick. It is impossible to predict the side effects that you will experience.

Benefits: This study is not being done to treat your cancer. Based on prior experience, the chance that you will feel better or live longer as a result of participating in this study is almost zero. This study is being done in the hope that it will provide information that will improve the treatment of people in the future.

CHAPTER 3-16

RESEARCH INVOLVING PRISONERS

ERNEST D. PRENTICE, BRUCE G. GORDON,
CHRISTOPHER J. KRATOCHVIL,
GAIL D. KOTULAK, AND ROBERT J. AMDUR

Research Involving Prisoners

In addition to the requirements for IRB approval that apply to all research, federal regulations require additional protections that are required for the IRB to approve research that involves prisoners:

- Any potential benefits from research participation are not coercive in the limited choice environment of the prison.

- The risks involved in the research are commensurate with risks that would be accepted by non-prisoner volunteers.

- The procedures for the selection of subjects within the prison are fair to all prisoners and immune from arbitrary intervention by prison authorities or prisoners.

- Participation in the research will have no effect on parole determinations.

Prisoners are considered a vulnerable subject population in need of additional protections, defined as follows in federal regulations:

"prisoner" means any individual involuntarily confined or detained in a penal institution. The term is intended to encompass individuals sentenced to such an institution under a criminal or civil statute as well as individuals detained in other facilities by virtue of statutes or commitment procedures which provide alternatives to criminal prosecution or incarceration in a penal institution, and individuals detained pending arraignment, trial, or sentencing.

This includes situations where a human subject becomes a prisoner after the research has commenced.

COMPOSITION OF THE IRB

According to federal regulations at 45 CFR 46.304(a)(b), the IRB reviewing prisoner research must be specially constituted. The board must include at least one member who is a prisoner or a prisoner representative with the appropriate background and experience to serve in that capacity. The IRB must be so constituted for all reviews of research involving prisoners, including initial review, continuing review, protocol amendments, and review of adverse events. If a human subject participating in an IRB-approved protocol becomes a prisoner after the research has begun, the protocol and consent document would need to be reviewed by the IRB again, with a prisoner representative present. Unless the IRB reapproves the research for inclusion of the prisoner(s), the newly incarcerated individual must be withdrawn from the study.

IRB APPROVAL CRITERIA FOR PRISONER RESEARCH

As with all other types of research, prisoner research must comply with the requirements of the general ethical codes and regulations that apply to research that does not involve prisoners. Basically, these requirements are that the risks to subjects must be minimized; risks to subjects are reasonable in relation to anticipated benefits; the selection of subjects is equitable; informed consent is obtained and appropriately documented; the research plan makes adequate provision for monitoring the data collected to ensure the safety of subjects; and there are adequate provisions to protect the privacy of subjects and to maintain the confidentiality of data.

In addition to these general requirements, federal regulations require additional protections for prisoners as research subjects by setting further conditions that must all be satisfied before the IRB can approve the study:

1. The research under review represents one of the categories of research permissible under 45 CFR 46.306(a)(2).

2. Any possible advantages accruing to the prisoner through his or her participation in the research, when compared to the general living conditions, medical care, quality of food, amenities and opportunity for earnings in the prison, are not of such a magnitude that his or her ability to weigh the risks of the research against the value of such advantages in the limited choice environment of the prison is impaired.

3. The risks involved in the research are commensurate with risks that would be accepted by nonprisoner volunteers.

4. The procedures for the selection of subjects within the prison are fair to all prisoners and immune from arbitrary intervention by prison authorities or prisoners. Unless the principal investigator provides to the board justification in writing for following some other procedures, control subjects must be selected randomly from the group of available prisoners who meet the characteristics needed for that particular research project.

5. The information is presented in language that is understandable to the subject population.

6. Adequate assurance exists that parole boards will not take into account a prisoner's participation in the

research in making decisions regarding parole, and each prisoner is clearly informed in advance that participation in the research will have no effect on his or her parole.

7. If the board finds that there may be a need for follow-up examination or care of participants after the end of their participation, adequate provision has been made for such examination or care, taking into account the varying lengths of individual prisoners' sentences, and for informing participants of this fact.

It should be noted that the last requirement is unclear in terms of how and to what extent the investigator, institution, or sponsor is responsible for providing care to both prisoners and parolees after their participation in research. Interpretation of this requirement is particularly problematic in clinical research on life-threatening illnesses such as cancer or AIDS where the patient is likely to need continued treatment, perhaps for a prolonged period and at considerable expense.

PROTECTION AT THE EXPENSE OF JUSTICE

The seven additional protections described above are obviously designed to protect the rights and welfare of prisoners who participate in research. Clearly, additional protection is needed. It is ironic, however, that these additional requirements also restrict the right of prisoners to participate in research. The result may be a paternalistic set of regulations that limit a prisoner's autonomy to decide to participate in and benefit from taking part in research. The Belmont principle of justice requires that both the benefits and burdens of research be distributed fairly. Also, by denying prisoners the ability to make a decision as to whether they want to participate in research, the Belmont principle of respect for persons may be violated. It is important for the IRB to consider these trade-offs when evaluating research that involves prisoners.

RESEARCH INVOLVING CHILDREN

ROBERT NELSON AND ROBERT J. AMDUR

Research Involving Children

Federal regulations permit the IRB to approve research involving children *only* if the research interventions or procedures fall into one of three categories:

1. Research involving "no greater than minimal risk to children."

2. Research involving an intervention or procedure presenting more than minimal risk to children that offers the "prospect of direct benefit" or may "contribute to the ... well-being" of the individual child. In addition, the risks must be justified by the anticipated benefit to the subjects and the relation of the anticipated benefit to the risk must be at least as favorable as that presented by available alternative approaches.

3. Research involving an intervention or procedure that presents only a "minor increase over minimal risk," yet does not offer any "prospect of direct benefit" or "contribute to the well-being" of the child. In addition, the intervention or procedure must present experiences to the subjects that are similar with their actual or expected situations, and likely yield generalizable knowledge of vital importance for understanding or ameliorating the child's disorder or condition.

THE ADDITIONAL SAFEGUARDS FOR CHILDREN IN RESEARCH

All of the ethical standards and regulatory requirements that apply to adults are required for the conduct of research involving children. In addition, 45CFR46 Subpart D of the DHHS regulations (and corresponding sections of 21CFR50 for FDA-regulated research) contain additional safeguards that the IRB must consider for research involving children. These safeguards follow two general approaches, based on the presence or absence of the prospect of direct benefit. First, when an intervention or procedure does not offer the prospect of direct benefit, the appropriate level of risk exposure is limited to either minimal risk (for any child) or a minor increase over minimal risk (for a child with the condition being studied). This restriction in allowable risk exposure corresponds to two categories of research involving children that allow for exposure to either "minimal risk" or a "minor increase over minimal risk." Second, when an intervention and/or procedure offers the prospect of direct benefit, the justification for acceptable risk exposure is limited to conditions approximating research equipoise. Thus the regulations permit the IRB to approve research involving children *only* if it falls into one of the following categories:

- **Research presenting "no greater than minimal risk to children."** The IRB determines that the level of risk is no greater than minimal, regardless of whether the research offers the prospect of direct benefit to the child. The level of risk that a child may be exposed to by interventions and/or procedures that do not offer the prospect of direct benefit is restricted to the level of risk that a child may be exposed to in the course of a child's everyday life. An intervention and/or procedure that offers the prospect of direct benefit yet presents only minimal risk is also approvable under this category.

- **Research involving an intervention or procedure presenting more than minimal risk to children that offers the "prospect of direct benefit" or may "contribute to the ... well-being" of the individual child.** The IRB may approve an intervention or procedure that offers the prospect of direct benefit to the individual child (or a monitoring procedure that is likely to contribute to the subject's well-being), and presents greater than minimal risk only if (1) the risk is justified by the anticipated benefit to the subjects and (2) the relation of the anticipated benefit to the risk is at least as favorable to the subjects as that presented by available alternative approaches. In effect, each arm of a study must have an appropriate risk/benefit balance, and the comparative therapeutic merits of each arm of a clinical trial should be balanced. The alternatives that must be considered include any available alternatives outside of the research study. The general principle is that a child should not be disadvantaged by entering a research study. A parent's decision to enroll a child in research should be similar to a decision to permit exposure to the risk and benefits of any nonresearch alternative.

- **Research involving an intervention or procedure that presents only a "minor increase over minimal risk," yet does not offer any "prospect of direct benefit" or "contribute to the well-being" of the child.** The limited conditions under which such research can be approved by an IRB include the following: (1) the risk represents only a minor increase over minimal risk; (2) the intervention or procedure presents experiences to subjects that are reasonably commensurate with those inherent in their actual or expected medical, dental, psychological, social, or educational situations; (3) the intervention or procedure is likely to yield generalizable knowledge about the subject's disorder or condition, which is of vital importance for the understanding or amelioration of the subject's disorder or condition.

All three categories require that adequate provisions are made for soliciting assent of the children and permission of their parents or guardians.

If an IRB cannot fit the research into one of these three categories, it must disapprove the research or refer it to a special review panel reporting to either the secretary of the DHHS or the FDA commissioner. However, before a research project can be referred to a federal panel, the local IRB must determine that "the research presents a reasonable opportunity to further the understanding, prevention, or alleviation of a serious problem affecting the health or welfare of children."

MINIMAL RISK AND A MINOR INCREASE OVER MINIMAL RISK

Guidelines under discussion at the federal level interpret minimal risk for research involving children to be that level of risk associated with the daily activities of a normal, healthy, average child. Risks include all harms, discomforts, indignities, embarrassments, and potential breaches of privacy and confidentiality associated with the research. Whether or not an intervention or procedure qualifies as minimal risk is not simply a statistical judgment, nor does it merely reflect that the risks associated with a procedure have been minimized. Conceptually, the minimal-risk standard defines a permissible level of risk in research as the socially (or normatively) allowable risks that parents generally permit their children to be exposed to in nonresearch situations.

Healthy children experience differing levels of risk in their daily lives. Indexing minimal risk to the socially (or normatively) allowable risks to which normal, average children are exposed routinely accounts for the differing risks experienced by children of different ages. However, the fact that some children may be exposed to differing levels of risk in the course of their daily lives may not justify greater risk exposure. If certain groups of children are routinely exposed to greater risks as part of their daily lives because of the circumstances in which they live, this level of increased risk ought *not* be interpreted as minimal risk just because it is part of the common experience of these otherwise healthy children. The phrase "ordinarily encountered in the daily life or during the performance of routine physical or psychological examinations or tests" is interpreted to mean an "equivalence of risk" rather than the procedure being one that is actually performed routinely. Thus a test or procedure that entails minimal risk is one for which the probability and magnitude of risk associated with the test or procedure is equivalent to and no greater than the risk of events ordinarily encountered in the daily life of a normal, healthy, average child, or the socially (or normatively) allowable risks parents permit their normal, healthy, average children to be exposed to in their ordinary lives.

A minor increase over minimal risk refers to those risks that are a little more than minimal and pose no significant threat to the child's health or well-being. While minimal risk is indexed to the risks encountered in the daily lives of normal, healthy, average children, the permissible level of risk associated with a minor increase over minimal should only be slightly more than that level and also commensurate with the risks of interventions or procedures having been experienced or expected to be experienced in the lives of children with a specific disorder or condition. Although some children may experience invasive procedures with considerable risk and discomfort during the care and treatment of a disease, this does not justify risks greater than a minor increase over minimal in a research study that provides no prospect of direct benefit to the individual subjects. In addition, this level of risk must be necessary in order to yield generalizable knowledge of vital importance for the understanding of the participants' disorder or condition.

DISORDER AND/OR CONDITION

The phrase "disorder and/or condition" refers to a characteristic of the group of potential research subjects, and implies that this characteristic can be understood more broadly than simply a specific disease or diagnostic category. Generally, the concept of disorder or condition relates to a specific characteristic that describes a group of children, such as a physical or social condition affecting children, or the risk of certain children developing a disease in the future based on diagnostic testing or physical examination. For example, prematurity, infancy, adolescence, poverty, living in a compromised physical environment, institutionalization, or having a genetic predisposition to future illness may be considered a disorder or condition in the context of an appropriate research protocol that, under the appropriate circumstances, warrants permissible research that presents levels of risk that are a minor increase over minimal levels without the prospect of direct benefit.

Approving Research Without Parental Permission

Federal regulations permit the IRB to approve research without the permission of a parent "if the IRB determines that a research protocol is designed for conditions or for a subject population for which ... permission is not a reasonable requirement to protect the subjects (for example, neglected or abused children), provided an appropriate mechanism for protecting the children who will participate as subjects in the research is substituted, and provided further that the waiver is not inconsistent with federal, state, or local law." For example, many pediatric IRBs will waive the requirement for parental permission for research using adolescent subjects that involves medical procedures and treatment that the adolescent can consent to without parental knowledge, such as use of contraceptives, treatment of sexually transmitted disease, treatment of alcohol and drug abuse, and so forth. However, the FDA does not allow the waiver of parental permission for research involving an FDA-regulated product.

CHILD ASSENT

Assent is defined as "a child's affirmative agreement to participate in research." A child's passive resignation to submit to an intervention or procedure must not be considered assent. The federal regulations do not specify any of the elements of informed assent and do not indicate an age at which assent ought to be possible. Clearly, assent needs to be "tailored to the level of comprehension of the prospective participants." An IRB is granted wide discretion in determining whether a child is capable of assenting and can waive the requirement for child assent under the following circumstances: if a child is not capable of assent; if the research offers a prospect of direct benefit not available outside of the research (thus falling under the scope of parental authority in overriding a child's desires); or given the same conditions under which parental permission can be waived. An IRB is granted wide discretion in determining whether and how a child's assent is documented.

PART 4

References for Additional Information

LIZ BANKERT AND ROBERT J. AMDUR

C H A P T E R   4-1

ETHICAL CODES

Nuremberg Code
Website:
http://ohrp.osophs.dhhs.gov/irb/irb_appendices.htm#j5

Belmont Report
Ethical Principles and Guidelines for the Protection of Human Subjects of Research
National Commission for the Protection of Human Subjects of Biomedical and Behavioral Research. April 18, 1979
Website: http://ohrp.osophs.dhhs.gov/humansubjects/guidance/belmont.htm

World Medical Association Declaration of Helsinki
Website: http://www.wma.net/e/policy/17-c_e.html

CHAPTER 4-2

U.S. GOVERNMENT REGULATIONS

Department of Health and Human Services
Office of Human Research Protection (OHRP)
Website: http://ohrp.osophs.dhhs.gov/

Protection of Human Subjects
45 Code of Federal Regulations Part 46
Website: http://www.med.umich.edu/irbmed/FederalDocuments/hhs/
HHS45CFR46.html

Revised Expedited Review Criteria (1998)
Website: http://ohrp.osophs.dhhs.gov/humansubjects/guidance/
expedited98.htm

Food and Drug Administration (FDA)
Website: http://www.fda.gov/

Protection of Human Subjects
21 Code of Federal Regulations Part 50
Website: http://www.access.gpo.gov/nara/cfr/waisidx_00/
21cfr50_00.html

Institutional Review Boards
21 Code of Federal Regulations Part 56
Website: http://www.access.gpo.gov/nara/cfr/waisidx_00/
21cfr56_00.html

Financial Disclosure by Clinical Investigators
21 Code of Federal Regulations Part 54
Website: http://www.access.gpo.gov/nara/cfr/waisidx_00/
21cfr54_00.html

Biologic Products: General
21 Code of Federal Regulations Part 600
Website: http://www.access.gpo.gov/nara/cfr/waisidx_00/
21cfr600_00.html

Investigational New Drug Application
21 Code of Federal Regulations Part 312
Website: http://www.access.gpo.gov/nara/cfr/waisidx_00/
21cfr312_00.html

Investigational Device Exemptions
21 Code of Federal Regulations Part 812
Website: http://www.access.gpo.gov/nara/cfr/waisidx_00/
21cfr812_00.html

Health Insurance Portability and Accountability Act (HIPAA)
Website: http://aspe.hhs.gov/admnsimp/

U.S. GOVERNMENT GUIDANCE/ RESOURCES

Office of Human Research Protection (OHRP): Dear Colleague Letters
Website: http://ohrp.osophs.dhhs.gov/dearcoll.htm

Office of Human Research Protection (OHRP): Guidance Topics by Subject
Website: http://ohrp.osophs.dhhs.gov/g-topics.htm

OHRP Compliance Activities: Common Findings and Guidance
Website: http://ohrp.osophs.gov/compovr.htm

FDA Information Sheets (1998 edition)
Guidance for Institutional Review Boards and Clinical Investigators
Website: http://www.fda.gov/oc/oha/IRB/toc.html

FDA Clinical Trials/Human Subjects Protection
Information for Health Professionals
Website: http://www.fda.gov/oc/oha/default.htm#clinical

National Bioethics Advisory Commission
Website: http://bioethics.gov/nbac.html

Office of Research Integrity
Website: http://ori.dhhs.gov/

Bioethics Resource on the Web—National Institutes of Health
Website: http://www.nih.gov/sigs/bioethics/

National Human Genome Research Institute
Ethical, Legal and Social Implications of Human Genetics Research
Website: http://www.nhgri.nih.gov/ELSI/

National Reference Center for Bioethics Literature—Kennedy Institute

Website: http://www.georgetown.edu/research/nrcbl/

Office of Biotechnology Activities—NIH

Website: http://www.nih.gov/od/oba/index.htm

INTERNATIONAL GUIDELINES

International Committee on Harmonization (ICH)
Good Clinical Practice Guidelines
Website: http://ncehr-cnerh.org/english/gcp

Council for International Organizations of Medical Sciences (CIOMS)
International Ethical Guidelines for Biomedical Research
Website: http://www.who.int/ina-ngo/ngo/ngo011.htm

National Council on Ethics in Human Research—Canada
Website: http://www.ncehr-cnerh.org/english/mstr_frm.html

C H A P T E R 4-5

BOOKS

Amdur, Robert J., and Bankert, Elizabeth (eds.). *Institutional Review Board: Management and Function.* Sudbury, MA: Jones and Bartlett, 2002.

Beauchamp, Tom L., and Childress, James F. *Principles of Biomedical Ethics,* 4th ed. New York: Oxford University Press, 1994.

Beauchamp, Tom L., Faden, Ruth R., Wallace, R. Jay, Jr., and Walters, LeRoy, eds. *Ethical Issues in Social Science Research.* Baltimore, MD: Johns Hopkins University Press, 1982.

Beauchamp, Tom L., and Childress, James F. *Principles of Biomedical Ethics,* 3rd ed. New York: Oxford University Press, 1989.

Beecher, Henry K. *Research and the Individual: Human Studies.* Boston: Little, Brown, 1970.

Brody, B.A. *The Ethics of Biomedical Research: An International Perspective.* New York: Oxford University Press, 1998.

Dunn, C., and Chadwick, G. *Protecting Study Volunteers in Research: A Manual for Investigative Sites.* Boston: Center Watch, 1999.

Faden, R. ed. *The Human Radiation Experiments.* New York: Oxford University Press, 1996.

Faden, Ruth R., and Beauchamp, Tom L. *A History of Theory of Informed Consent.* New York: Oxford University Press, 1986.

Freund, Paul A., ed. *Experimentation with Human Subjects.* New York: George Braziller, 1970.

Jonsen, Veatch, Walters. *Source Book in Bioethics: A Documentary History.* Washington: Georgetown University Press, 1998.

Katz, Jay, with the assistance of Alexander Morgan Capron and Eleanor Swift Glass. *Experimentation with Human Beings: The Authority of the Investigator, Subject, Professions, and State in the Human Experimentation Process.* New York: Russell Sage Foundation, 1972.

Levine, R.J. *The Ethics and Regulation of Clinical Research,* 2nd ed. New Haven: Yale University Press, 1988.

Penslar, R.L. *Research Ethics: Cases and Materials.* Bloomington: Indiana University Press, 1995.

Protecting Human Research Subjects: Institutional Review Board Guidebook. Bethesda, MD: Office for Protection from Research Risks, 1993.

Russell-Einhorn, M., ed. *IRB Reference Book.* Washington: Price Waterhouse Coopers, LLP, 2000.

Sieber, Joan E. *Planning Ethically Responsible Research: A Guide for Students and Internal Review Boards.* Applied Social Research Methods Series, vol. 31. Newbury Park, CA: Sage Publications, 1992.

Sieber, Joan E., ed. *The Ethics of Social Research: Surveys and Experiments.* New York: Springer-Verlag, 1982.

Sieber, Joan E., ed. *The Ethics of Social Research: Fieldwork, Regulation, and Publication.* New York: Springer-Verlag, 1982.

Sugarman, Mastroianni, Kahn. *Ethics of Research with Human Subjects: Selected Policies and References.* Frederick, MD: University Publishing Group, 1998.

Vanderpool, H.Y. *The Ethics of Research Involving Human Subjects.* Frederick, MD: University Publishing Group, 1996.

Veatch, Robert M. *Medical Ethics.* Boston: Jones and Bartlett, 1989.

PERIODICALS AND THE IRB FORUM

ARENA Newsletter
Applied Research Ethics in Medicine and Research
http://140.239.168.132/arena.html

Bulletin of Medical Ethics
Dr. Richard Nicholson, Editor
E-mail: bulletin_of_medical_ethics@compuserve.com

The Hastings Center
Website: http://www.thehastingscenter.org/

Hastings Center Report
Website: http://www.thehastingscenter.org/publications.htm

IRB: A Review of Human Subjects Research
Website: http://www.thehastingscenter.org/publications.htm

Human Research Report
Website: http://www.humansubjects.com/

Kennedy Institute of Ethics Journal
Website: http://muse.jhu.edu/journals/kennedy_institute_of_
ethics_journal/

Research Practitioner
Website: http://www.researchpractice.com/rp_about.shtml

The IRB Forum (previously MCWIRB)
The IRB Forum (previously called MCWIRB) promotes the
discussion of ethical, regulatory and policy concerns with
human subjects research.
Website: http://www.irbforum.org/

CHAPTER 4-7

VIDEO RECORDINGS

Columbia University Seminars on Media and Society, in association with WNET New York. *The Human Experiment.* Produced by Betsy Miller and Martha Elliot. Annenberg: CPB Project, 1989.

National Library of Medicine. *Evolving Concern: Protection of Human Subjects.* Produced for the U.S. National Institutes of Health and the U.S. Food and Drug Administration. Bethesda, MD: National Institutes of Health, Office for the Protection from Research Risks, 1986.

National Library of Medicine. *The Belmont Report: Basic Ethical Principles and the Application.* Produced for the U.S. National Institutes of Health and the U.S. Food and Drug Administration. Bethesda, MD: National Institutes of Health, Office for the Protection from Research Risks, 1986.

National Library of Medicine. *Balancing Society's Mandates: IRB Review Criteria.* Produced for the U.S. National Institutes of Health and the U.S. Food and Drug Administration. Bethesda, MD: National Institutes of Health, Office for the Protection from Research Risks, 1986.

ORGANIZATIONS

American Society of Law, Medicine, and Ethics (ASLME)
Website: http://www.aslme.org/

Applied Research Ethics National Association (ARENA)
Website: http://140.239.168.132/arena.html

CenterWatch Clinical Trials
Website: http://www.centerwatch.com

Drug Information Association (DIA)
Website: http://www.diahome.org

National Association of IRB Managers (NIAM)
Website: http://www.naim.org

Public Responsibility in Medicine and Research (PRIM&R)
Website: http://www.primr.org